Cognitive-Constructivist Psychotherapy with Children and Adolescents

Cognitive-Constructivist Psychotherapy with Children and Adolescents

Tammie Ronen
The Bob Shapell School of Social Work
Tel Aviv University
Tel Aviv, Israel

Kluwer Academic / Plenum Publishers
New York, Boston, Dordrecht, London, Moscow

Library of Congress Cataloging-in-Publication Data

Ronen, Tammie
Cognitive-constructivist psychotherapy with children and adolescents/by Tammie Ronen.
p. ; cm.
Includes bibliographical references and index.
ISBN 0-306-47367-4
1. Cognitive therapy for children—Case studies. 2. Cognitive therapy for teenagers—Case studies. 3. Constructionism (Psychology) 4. Child psychotherapy—Case studies. 5. Adolescent psychotherapy—Case studies. I. Title.
[DNLM: 1. Cognitive Therapy—Adolescence—Case Report. 2. Cognitive Therapy—Child—Case Report. 3. Mental Disorders—therapy—Adolescence—Case Report. 4. Mental Disorders—therapy—Child—Case Report. WS 350.6 R772ca 2002]
RJ505.C63 R658 2002
618.92′89142—dc21

2002028687

ISBN 0-306-47367-4

233 Spring Street, New York, New York 10013

http://www.wkap.nl/

10 9 8 7 6 5 4 3 2 1

A C.I.P. record for this book is available from the Library of Congress

Printed in the United States of America

To my husband, Michael Rosenbaum, who brought back happiness, joy, and creativity into my personal as well as my professional life, and became a real partner to each moment and each area of my being.

Foreword

In an ideal training program for mental health professionals, every apprentice would be asked to spend time with two groups of people: children and dying elders. Both are among our most instructive teachers. The poet Kahlil Gibran liked to remind us that we should be wary of religions that do not laugh, philosophies that do not cry, and any perspective that does not bow to the inherent beauty of the child. There are many ways of conceptualizing therapeutic work with a child, of course. I believe that the most adequate of these frameworks bespeak a capacity to honor each child's current grasp of their worlds and their options within it. If a therapist knows how to work with a child—how to let go of words as the only way to communicate, how to trust in an unfolding nowness, how to dance with the edges of hope and fear—then that therapist is better prepared to work with adults.

The other end of the spectrum—working with dying elders—may seem disconnected, but I believe that it involves and refines similar skills. It also involves learning to be genuinely "with" another person, often without words, and to trust that the being together in and of itself is a gesture of life. Elders have often paid high and painful prices for lessons about life—lessons that include insights about what is really important. Hospice workers have noted that the most frequently voiced regrets on our deathbeds are primarily regrets about paths not taken and life experiences not risked. Indeed, I think it fair to also say that dying elders often remind us to honor the child in us at every age.

Some of my most precious memories as a human being—far beneath and beyond my occasional role as a helping professional—have been formed on playgrounds and in hospices, often with either tiny and young or weathered and old hands holding my own. I am still learning, of course, but those lessons have consistently highlighted the importance of being an engaged participant.

In an ideal training program for mental health professionals, there would be mentors like Tammie Ronen. She is a rare and precious specimen who sees and empowers the rarity, the preciousness, and the power of the people with whom she works. This marvelous book is about helping children. Tammie is one of the most creative child therapists in the world. This volume is not only a testament to her work but, more importantly, to the processes of adapting and developing which she aspires to serve.

When I think of Tammie Ronen, I am reminded of a line once offered by anthropologist Ashley Montagu. He was speaking about the significance of life-long flexibility, openness to experience, and playfulness. Montagu suggested that our goal in life should be "to die as young as possible as late as we can." By the word "young," of course, he meant child-like. His thesis was that our child-like capacities are our most valuable assets in all adaptation, learning, and development. Our capacities for playfulness, imagination, and creativity are more than life phase peculiarities. They are the heart of our "plasticity"—the engines of human change processes.

This book is a wonderful and welcome illustration of a constructive approach to the treatment of troubled children. Constructivism is a contemporary expression of an appreciation that embraces both ancient and modern insights into the patterns and processes of human experiencing. Fundamentally developmental in orientation, constructivism views each individual as a uniquely unfolding expression of life. Our personal senses of identity develop within contexts of relationships. Selves cannot be separated from systems or vice-versa. Each of us (and all others) can be understood only as active participants in the creation of meaning in our lives. Meaning is, in fact, relational. As Tammie and her clients so powerfully illustrate, meaning is an ever-unfolding relationship (with oneself, with one's feelings and thoughts, with other people and the world). We feel and act and think in an integrative holism of being. Children teach us that, often far more powerfully than elders.

The unique form of work that Tammie Ronen writes about in this book is a valuable expression of the wisdom of working simultaneously inside, outside, and alongside our clients. She combines an appreciation for the subjective world of the child with respect for environmental contexts, real-life demands, and developmental histories. Moreover, her work with children emphasizes that creativity is central to adaptation. Using methods that range from movement and drawing to imagination and play, she shows how children can be helped to find and express their own powers as active agents in their own lives.

This book offers a new way of conceptualizing therapeutic work with children. It also offers many examples of new ways of being and working as a therapist. I hope that it will inspire many to imagine, explore, and create in their own ways.

MICHAEL MAHONEY

Acknowledgments

This book is an outcome of many years of discussions with my dearest friend and colleague, Michael Mahoney. While seeing each other at conferences and professional meetings, while talking with each other between courses in restaurants, and even while dancing and joking at parties, we have shared our experiences of the treatment process and its techniques and strategies. It has taken quite some time for Michael Mahoney's imploring to sink in: that I should take time out from my busy schedule of writing about theory and research and should begin writing about my real work, the unique way in which I view and treat children. I will always be grateful for his persistence that led to the writing of this volume.

Writing a book is a creative process that consolidates thoughts as well as emotions, discussions, memories, images, and knowledge based on working for many years with many people. It is a pleasant obligation to express my appreciation to those who have been instrumental in helping bring this work to fruition.

First of all, my deepest thanks go to my clients, the children and adolescents. Most of what I do, I have learned from them. They challenged me by asking, demanding, and proposing techniques and strategies. They taught me to open my ears and eyes and listen to their wishes, words, and needs.

The case studies in this volume all describe children whom I have been treating at my private clinic during the last few years. The reports of these cases are true to these remarkable children's own words and the actual events transpiring during treatment; however, to honor their dignity and their secrets, I made changes in these youngsters' names, ages, and demographic components.

I am also indebted to my university students, whose inexhaustible curiosity and unrelenting insistence that I describe in detail the "how to do what" of child therapy, induced me to record my clinical work via audiotape and videotape and to document some of the cases for teaching purposes.

To my friends and colleagues at the Bob Shapell School of Social Work, who enabled me to finance the editing of this book, I am very grateful.

The chapter relating to opposition defiant disorder was supported by grants to our university research clinic from the Ashalim Organization for Youth at Risk and their Families and from the Pratt Foundation. The *Empowering Children and Adolescents for Self-Control Research Clinic* treats and studies children with aggressive behavior. I extend my appreciation to them.

And last but not least, I want to thank my editor, Dee B. Ankonina. Dee has edited all of my professional writing up to now and hopefully will continue to do so in the future, but also has become a good friend with whom to share, discuss, and consult.

Contents

Introduction

One set of parents I counseled told me that their child was like a moving target. Whenever they thought they had reached him, he was already moving onward to somewhere else, and they kept running after him, trying to understand him and to give him what he needed, without success. I think this is a good metaphor for the area of child psychotherapy in general. The field of child and adolescent therapy has grown remarkably over the last 30 years. New assessment tools, new studies on child development, and new techniques and strategies have come to the aid of the therapist. Over a decade ago, Kazdin (1988a) counted 230 different therapeutic techniques directed toward childhood and adolescence. This abundance opens up greater choices but does not necessarily provide answers to the continual debates about what can best benefit children and what is the best way to treat children and adolescents.

Child psychotherapy was traditionally based on dynamic play therapy, believing that children are too young to understand, analyze, or talk about their disorders and therefore need to play out their concerns and problems.

Behavior therapy, on the other hand, was based on learning processes and therefore attempted to condition children to adopt new behaviors. Yet this approach neglected the role of emotions, believing that if a behavior changed, the emotions and thoughts would follow it.

Cognitive therapy with children is still in the first stage of struggling to prove its efficacy for children. Questions continue to be raised as to whether children can benefit from cognitive therapy, to what extent, at what ages, and via which techniques.

There is still very limited knowledge and literature on constructivist therapy with children. Most of the knowledge is taken from constructivist therapy with adults. This therapeutic approach appears promising, but the need remains to develop specific assessment and treatment tools for children.

The traditional position of child and adolescent therapy is one of great dichotomies: between direct and indirect therapy with children (cognitive or behavior versus dynamic, respectively) as well as between verbal and nonverbal techniques with children (i.e. conversation or discussion versus play, art, music, or movement). During the last decade, changes have emerged in psychotherapy research and treatment. Especially notable has been the appearance of studies in the areas of human change processes (Mahoney, 1991), interpersonal processes (Safran & Segal, 1990), and the role of emotion in psychotherapy (Greenberg & Safran, 1987). Those studies have enabled the use of more experimental and experiential techniques. Also, they focused on the need to integrate emotions and relationships into the basically rational cognitive treatment model. This blend has contributed considerably to the treatment of disorders in childhood and adolescence, in general, and in the area of cognitive therapy, in particular.

In this book, I maintain a theoretical orientation that espouses a cognitive-developmental approach that integrates constructivist concepts and techniques. Yet, I propose that its application can consolidate a variety of traditional and innovative techniques, methods, and strategies to facilitate change in children. Indirect nonverbal tools, for example, can be applied to cognitive therapy just as easily as they fit into traditional psychodynamic therapy. The real issue is not the use or selection of specific techniques, but rather the creative thinking and open attitude that can help the therapist transform his or her therapeutic goals into those modes of intervention best suited to the individual child's needs.

I would like to give a few examples to illustrate what I mean. Several years ago, while touring a nature reserve in southern Israel, I happened upon a young blond boy, about the age of three, who was crying, kicking, and shouting while his young parents stood helpless and embarrassed a few feet away. I overheard that the boy had refused to continue walking, fearing that a snake might bite him. Apparently, none of the parents' explanations, persuasions, or threats was sufficient to make him continue. In terms of cognitive–constructivist theory, it was the boy's way of thinking (his construction) that made him fear the snake, and only by changing the "meaning making" of the event could he cope with it. Having no time for therapy (nor had anyone sought my help), I simply asked the little boy who the snake was afraid of. Without hesitation, he said, "A lion." "Could you be a lion?" I asked. "Sure," he said. He got down on all fours as if he were a lion, made a frightening face, and started moving forward. He had changed the meaning of the situation from "I'm scared! The snake will bite me!" to "The snake will stay away because the lion is even more scary." Momentarily, the problem was over, and the child continued walking.

Another case is that of a 5-year-old boy whose parents brought him to a community mental health center where I was working. The child was suffering from daytime encopresis (soiling his pants). In describing the boy's history, his parents insisted that he was not a particularly fearful child, and that he had no special problems other than his refusal to sit on the toilet and his soiling of his pants. However, at a time when there was no progress in therapy, I suggested that the boy come with me to the bathroom. As we gradually approached the door, he edged closer and closer to me. As I opened the door, he jumped on me, pale, shaking, and clinging to me tightly. He started to cry, and I understood from him that he was afraid of a big monster. Later on, he told me that in his kindergarten the children said there was a monster living inside the toilet. That monster, he was told, would come out whenever someone emptied himself or herself, because the feces were the monster's food. For the next few treatment sessions, I brought bread, and we entered the bathroom together, trying to feed the creature and flush the water down. When no monster came out, slowly the boy started relaxing. Following this intervention, his soiling began to decrease and eventually disappeared.

In both cases, my objective was to change the child's way of looking at the event, and thereby changing his way of thinking and his construction of an event, in order to help the child cope better. These examples illustrate how much faster and more effective it can be with young children to use metaphors or games. It also highlights the need to view the problem from their own perspective with their own language. Taking the children's viewpoint is much more efficient than trying to convince them that they are mistaken or illogical, or to wait until children initiate important issues spontaneously in play.

This book aims to mobilize the therapist's creative thinking within cognitive–constructivist theory, while emphasizing the importance of finding the individual meaning making for each child. Verbal therapy, play therapy, games, music, and whatever suits the particular client's meaning making process, are the treatments of choice. To foster the reader's understanding of this approach, I will present case studies where I treated different childhood and adolescent disorders by adapting various techniques to each child's needs.

Before expounding on these issues, I would like to make one more important comment. The complexity of child therapy begins with the definition of whom we call a "child" and what we consider the age limits of childhood. This book refers to children as well as adolescents, because for me (unlike many others), adolescence is a unique yet an integral part of childhood. Many of the characteristics of childhood—rapid change, unique language, unique thinking style, gaps between chronological, emotional, and cognitive age, etc.—characterize adolescence as well. Therefore, while talking about children, I relate to the whole spectrum of childhood, from birth up until the entrance into adulthood.

And, finally, as anyone intervening with children knows, the treatment process is a complex, challenging, and interesting one. I have decided to take up the challenge and write this book about my clients. The book presents my clinical approach to child therapy, and the techniques I have found helpful in this ever-changing and rewarding work. I hope that this book succeeds in communicating to my readers what I feel and do when undertaking the treatment of children who are suffering.

OVERVIEW

This book offers theory, an intervention model, clinical illustrations, and conclusions leading to practical guidelines, comprising four parts. The first part reviews literature and provides a theoretical foundation. The second part builds on the first, offers guidelines for making decisions about children while designing the intervention process, and proposes a self-control intervention model. The third part discusses specific childhood disorders and illustrates my approach through case studies. The fourth part offers some thoughts about the entire process of change, in particular as a function of the therapeutic relationship and the therapist's own flexibility and creativity.

The theoretical foundation, presented in Part I, is grounded in three major theoretical domains. First, the unique developmental features typifying childhood are discussed, in order to help therapists identify those elements characteristic of children necessitating special consideration when designing interventions (e.g. age, gender, cognitive and emotional development, motivation, personal style and interests, the normative basis for childhood disorders, spontaneous change and recovery, etc.). Next, the theoretical foundation underlying cognitive–constructivist interventions is reviewed and applied to the specific nature of working with children and adolescents. Finally, conceptual aspects of tapping one's creative human capacities are presented, highlighting the importance of psychotherapists' creative and flexible implementation of a range of techniques in child intervention. These three domains aim to provide a solid framework to underlie child clinical intervention. The section also aims at fostering therapists' ability to creatively design a unique intervention for each individual child. This intervention should be based on the child's specific needs (e.g. developmental characteristics, linguistic idiosyncrasies, and personal interests) as well as on the unique nature of the child's particular disorder, with a reliance on cognitive–constructivist principles and creative methods.

Part II is my own interpretation of Part I, where I combine these three issues into guidelines for the therapist regarding decision making in child cognitive–constructivist therapy (Chapter 4). Then, Chapter 5 presents my self-control intervention model for changing children's behavior as well as their thoughts and feelings, based on the consolidation of cognitive–constructivist therapy with developmental considerations and creative thinking.

Part III of the book demonstrates the application of the proposed approach through a series of case studies representing a large range of self-control intervention techniques as adapted to different ages and cognitive levels. The two cases presented for treating young children and supervising their parents, through the use of drawing, play, and movement techniques, include one child with a case of anxiety and phobia, and another with selective mutism. The two cases of children in middle childhood, who were treated using verbal therapy, constructs, and charting, include an abused child and another with psychosomatic pain. The three cases of adolescents combine verbal discussion and techniques with metaphors and imagery training. One case relates to enuresis, one describes a boy with oppositional defiant disorder, and the third child was treated for depression.

A brief review of the literature dealing with the characteristics of each disorder is presented prior to the description of the cognitive–constructivist treatment process developed for each of these children that integrates verbal and nonverbal, direct and indirect methods.

Part IV presents a summary and some conclusions related to the role of therapeutic relationships in cognitive constructivist therapy with children, emphasizing the importance of creative techniques in treatment. This fourth part integrates the cognitive–constructivist therapy with creative intervention for children and adolescents. In the epilogue, I suggest how professional training must incorporate opportunities for each of us as therapists to find and experience the creative child within.

I hope this book will be helpful in presenting new ideas to therapists and in challenging clinicians both to dare to treat children and also to dare to use new modes of intervention that will facilitate the treatment process.

TAMMIE RONEN

I

Theoretical Ground for Cognitive–Constructivist Psychotherapy with Children and Adolescents

1

The Unique Nature of Child Psychotherapy

Developmental components are an integral part of making decisions about children's therapy throughout the entire process of intervention (Mash & Dozois, 1996). At different ages and stages of development and differentially for boys and girls, specific processes and opportunities may emerge, in domains such as cognitive comprehension, exposure to new experiences, establishing relationships, perceiving and expressing emotions, and more (Ronen, 1997a,b). A multitude of etiological models and treatment approaches have been proposed to explain and remediate psychopathology in children (Mash & Dozois, 1996). At the same time, research suggests that a diversity of techniques is needed in order to achieve change, each one suiting children at different cognitive stages and transition periods, and depending on the specific problem areas (Kazdin, 1994b).

In contrast with traditional therapists, cognitive behavior therapists stress that clients are not treated because of their disorders but because of the way they cope with these disorders (Kanfer & Schefft, 1988). This is especially true with children, who experience emotional and behavioral disturbances as a natural, integral part of their normal developmental processes. This normative basis for common childhood phenomena (e.g. fears and anxieties, enuresis, aggressiveness, learning difficulties, obsessive-compulsive rituals, social deficits, eating problems) hinders the differentiation between a normal developmental reaction and a behavioral dysfunction. Kazdin (1988a) stated that only a small proportion of children in need will be referred to therapy and that referred children do not necessarily comprise that group in greatest need. As the next section will show, a number of decisive issues characterize child therapy and differentiate it from that of adults.

THE COMPLEXITY OF CHILD THERAPY

The area of child psychotherapy is uniquely complex and differs from adult therapy in many facets throughout all its stages, beginning with assessment, continuing with the design of the treatment setting and conducting the intervention process, and concluding with the evaluation and maintenance of the treatment's outcome. The diagnostic stage of child therapy requires taking into account the constant changes and incongruencies typifying the childhood years on the one hand, and the need to adapt treatments to children's particular features, such as thinking patterns, dependence on adults, and use of language, on the other. Several major characteristics unique to childhood should be considered, particularly during the assessment process.

The Normal Basis of Most Childhood Disorders

Epidemiological studies and large-scale surveys indicate that emotional and behavioral problems are quite common among children (e.g. Kazdin, 1994b). Social changes and conditions may place children at increasingly greater risk for the development of disorders and also for the development of more severe problems at younger ages (Mash & Dozois, 1996). However, the extent to which such problems signify severe psychopathology is much lower (Campbell, 1990). The majority of childhood disorders begin as developmentally normal problems. They become deviant in one of two ways (Mash & Terdal, 1988; Ronen, 1997b): Either they persist longer than expected, as when bedwetting becomes diagnosed as enuresis, or they increase, instead of decrease, in frequency, as when sleep problems evolve into sleep terror disorder. To determine when a behavior previously considered normal should be viewed as maladaptive, age criteria are typically employed, despite unequivocal cut-off ages.

Developmental Incongruities

Discrepancies are prevalent between children's chronological age and their emotional, cognitive, and behavioral ages (Ronen, 1997b; Sahler & McAnarney, 1981). For example, the age-appropriate emotional maturity of a highly intelligent 6-year-old boy may be incongruous with his environment's expectations, based on his precocious cognitive and academic performance, leading to confusion and dissatisfaction from his behavior. Such gaps create a challenge for therapists in their attempt to assess and diagnose an individual child referred to therapy, meriting specific attention.

Spontaneous Developmental Changes

Assessing children who are referred to therapy is made complex by the temporary nature of many problematic behaviors during childhood. Wenar (1982) contended that when problems occur in children, the effect can best be described as "normal development gone awry." Many researchers (e.g. Doleys, 1977; Shirk & Russel, 1996) have asserted that a large proportion of problematic children will resolve their problems even without intervention, considering that, in children, spontaneous recovery is the norm. What seemed to be a problem yesterday is not necessarily what disturbs a child today. He or she may quickly show mastery, with little evidence that the challenge was other than momentary. Other studies have emphasized the fact that children exhibit transient difficulties while struggling to deal with the challenges of normal development (Mash & Barkley, 1996; Schaffer, 1996). Children's constant and rapid changes in motoric, emotional, and cognitive skills can be at the root of behavioral and emotional disturbances such as impulsivity in early childhood, sleep disorders in middle childhood, or mood shifts and anger during adolescence. It is up to the diagnostician to ascertain if the identified symptoms in fact warrant treatment, by utilizing knowledge about spontaneous recovery for this specific problem area as well as information on the pace and progression of this particular child's problem.

Environmental Variability in Functioning

The complexity of common child referrals to therapy includes problems in several components: the personal functioning of the child (e.g. enuresis, tics, stuttering, anorexia, trichotillomania); the child's relationships with the immediate adult environment such as school and family (e.g. disobedience, aggression, negativism); or the child's peer relations (e.g. interpersonal skill deficits, social withdrawal, peer rejection) (Achenbach, 1985; Hughes, 1993; Kazdin, 1988a). Children very often function differently in the significant settings in their lives, that is, in the home, classroom, and peer group. A child can evidence an undesired behavior only at home or in one specific classroom, or at recess. These disparities make it difficult to determine whether children demonstrate specific deficits or whether an environment has conditioned them and has provided positive reinforcement to certain unwanted behaviors. Such a differentiation is crucial within a comprehensive assessment process, in order to reach a decision of whether it is the child or the environment that should be the target of intervention (Kazdin, 1988a).

External Motivation for Referral

Adults, rather than the children themselves, are most often those who bring the youngsters for therapeutic assessment. Consequently, the therapist must be sensitive to the prevalent incongruity between what disturbs children and what disturbs their parents and teachers. Expressing the common wish to help children change their behavior (Kratochwill & Morris, 1993), adults who bring children to treatment do so primarily because of behavioral problems that disturb the surrounding adult population. Such acting-out or "undercontrolled" problems include disobedience, aggressiveness, and impulsiveness. Yet, those behaviors do not necessarily disturb the children as much as the acting-in or "overcontrolled" disorders such as depression, anxiety, or loneliness, which are less often seen by clinicians and are often in great need of treatment (Mash & Terdal, 1988; Ronen, 1993b,c, 1995, 1997b). Even when children who were victims of abuse or neglect at the hands of adults are referred, the presented behavior is typically of an acting-out nature that disturbs adults.

Disparities Between Information Sources

A related area unique to children's assessment and intervention is the complexity involved in obtaining reliable information from the sources available to the clinician: the child, parents, teachers, peers, and direct observation (Achenbach, 1985; Ronen, 1997b). Research has demonstrated that each of these sources can provide reliable information in some areas, while a reliance on any one source alone may provide an incomplete or biased picture.

Direct assessment of the child through verbal interviews, self-report questionnaires, and formal diagnostic testing is a crucial source of reliable information on the child's own outlook toward inner feelings, self-esteem, and perceptions of the environment. Children's self-reports of acting-in behaviors (i.e. overcontrolled or internalizing behaviors such as depression and fears) have been shown to be more reliable than their parents' reports in this area (Achenbach, 1993; Kazdin, 1988a,b). In contrast, children's self-reports are not as reliable a source regarding their own acting-out, undercontrolled, or externalizing behaviors such as disruptiveness and oppositional defiant disorders, in comparison with parental reports of such conduct.

Direct observation helps the therapist to become acquainted with the child and his or her behavior within the child's natural environment. It reduces the dependency on parents' memories or subjective interpretations and on other misleading factors. However, proponents of the observation method claim that the child's natural behavior differs in his or her various environmental settings, rendering only one observation in one setting insufficient. Several observations may therefore be required.

Parents have traditionally been a chief source of information for the therapist at referral (Hughes, 1993). Yet, parents tend to emphasize their children's disruptive, undercontrolled behaviors like aggression, disobedience, and negativism. At the same time, they underestimate their children's emotional, overcontrolled problems such as loneliness, anxiety, and depression (Hodges et al., 1990). Based on this tendency among parents, it is suggested that parents should be considered a wellhead of data on the former but only a supplementary source of information on the latter.

Teachers comprise an important source of information on their students' academic difficulties, social adjustment within the peer context, and behavior in the classroom (e.g. disobedience, hyperactivity). However, as is the case for parents, teacher reports demonstrate a low reliability with regard to children's emotional, overcontrolled disorders. Peer reports and sociometric questionnaires may provide additional data on children's social functioning.

The need is obvious for therapists to integrate diverse sources of information (and diagnostic tools) into their assessment procedures. While doing so, therapists should include: the child, to provide his or her own subjective perspective; the parents, as the authority on the child within the family; and the teacher and peers, to add knowledge concerning the child relative to his or her age and sex group (Shirk & Russell, 1996).

Linguistic and Cognitive Features and Personal Style

Several features depicting different stages of development pose a challenge for therapists during the assessment process. Children's usage of verbal language is not fully developed, restricting their verbal understanding and expressiveness. Most significantly, their concrete and very subjective perception of the world colors their responses to standard assessment procedures in ways that are not always sufficiently acknowledged. Unlike adults, whose responses to such procedures vary but should fall within expected parameters, children have not fully undergone socialization processes. They remain steeped in their familial and cultural customs and perceptions, and have not yet gained the ability to clearly differentiate reality from imagination.

A variety of methods available to child practitioners does exist, not only with regard to treatment methods but also in diagnostic techniques for evaluating children's problems. Yet the large majority of nonverbal, unmediated diagnostic and therapeutic tools such as drawing, free association, and storytelling depend on the therapist's individual interpretation of the child's responses. Although the reliability or validity of these interpretations cannot be substantiated, the need to conduct a deeper inquiry into the child's personal attributions and thinking processes should be maintained as an important principle during assessment. An awareness of a specific child's interests, hobbies, individual style, habits, attitudes, language, way of thinking, and social and cultural context can be crucial in differentiating between pathological responses and normal ones. Standard testing procedures, unfortunately, rarely incorporate the children's own explanations regarding their specific responses to test questions (Kazdin, 1988a; Mash & Terdal, 1988).

This chapter will now elaborate on several developmental features that should be taken into account by therapists working with children: gender, cognitive and emotional level, motivation, and idiosyncratic style.

GENDER AS A COMPONENT TO BE CONSIDERED

Gender constitutes an important component while assessing and treating children (Ronen, 1998a). Gender differences may be explained by several factors, such as social norms or a variation in maturation processes. On the one hand, girls as a group mature more quickly than boys; so one can expect that girls will exhibit fewer disorders with an important developmental component. On the other hand, role taking influences girls by allowing them to talk more freely about anxieties and fears than do boys; thus, reports of anxiety are usually higher among girls (Kazdin, 1988a; Ronen, 1998a).

The development of sexual identity among children emerges in three stages. First, children develop gender identity (categorizing themselves as male or female). Then, gender stability emerges (an awareness that usually boys grow up to be men and girls grow up to be women); and, finally, gender consistency is attained (the recognition of the gender group to which the child belongs and an understanding of its implications) (Kohlberg & Ullian, 1974).

Gender influences development and has an impact on the assessment of behavioral dysfunction by influencing social expectations. For example, in general, patterns of play and social relations differ among boys and girls. School-aged girls tend to be tied more to one or two significant friends of their own age and sex, whereas boys tend to play in large same-sex groups. Girls find it more difficult to make new friends than do boys (Raviv et al., 1990). The fact that sex mediates social relationships and to some degree predicts social adjustment to new environments (Raviv et al., 1990) also contributes to assessment and intervention processes. Gender has a greater influence as children grow up and enter the adolescent stage, acquiring specific sex roles; studies point to greater differences between the sexes as children mature.

While treating children, gender is an important consideration. For example, during the assessment process, girls are often more receptive to an invitation to draw than are boys. A diagnosis may also differ for boys and girls; for example, assessing a boy as anorexic (which is a significantly more common diagnosis among girls) may point to a more severe disorder. Similarly, because aggression is more frequently seen among boys, perhaps a girl who presents severe aggressive behavior should be assessed more carefully. During intervention, girls often cooperate better with play therapy than boys, especially at preadolescence. Also, in late adolescence when sex identity and social skills are especially important, 16–17-year-old male adolescents often respond better to a male therapist than to a female one. Gender may also come into play in making decisions about group intervention; at certain ages children do not respond well to heterogeneous groups, whereas in adolescence a combination of boys and girls in the same group can contribute to motivation.

THE IMPACT OF CHILDREN'S COGNITIVE LEVEL

A critical issue related to young children in therapy is that of their cognitive functioning. Many therapists believe that it is impossible to treat young children because they have not mastered cognitive abilities in the areas of verbal expression, abstraction, and concentration. The truth is that, at each age and stage, children can be treated if only the therapist designs intervention strategies and methods in line with the child's cognitive developmental sophistication (Bierman & Furman, 1984; Knell, 1993). Being aware of the child's cognitive level, strengths, and limitations enables the therapist to design the treatment process and techniques in a way that will appropriately meet the child's developmental needs (Knell, 1993). For example, younger children's appreciation of time is limited; therefore, distant goals and long-term benefits are incomprehensible, whereas short-term gratification and displeasure are vivid in comparison, shaping the design of treatment objectives.

Piaget's (1924) classification of children's cognitive development into four stages can serve as a general guideline for therapeutic planning. In the sensorimotor stage (birth to 2 years), children have limited cognitive and language skills and explore their environment predominantly through sensory and motoric means. Therapy during this stage is thus necessarily directed toward the child's environment. In the pre-operational stage (3–5 years), children evidence rapid conceptual and language development, and thinking becomes symbolic. The child can be a good candidate for individual therapy as long as the therapist remembers to use symbolic language and concrete concepts, and to appeal to the child's illogical, subjective way of thinking. "Experiential" therapy, using drawing, painting, music, dancing, and so on could best suit the child's ability to learn. In the concrete operational stage (6–11 years), children's thinking remains concrete and egocentric, yet abstract concepts can be understood in a limited way, and rapid academic learning occurs. Verbal therapy can now easily be applied, if based on the child's day-to-day life and experiences, not on universal concepts, notions, and rational arguments. In the abstract or formal operational stage (from age 12), preadolescents and adolescents develop an adult-like way of thinking, including dealing with abstract and holistic concepts. Verbal therapy can now be seen as an interesting challenge; whereas nonverbal therapy may even be insulting to the young person who wishes to be treated like an adult.

It is up to the therapist to determine the child's individual learning pace and style, and ability to generalize learned material. Through careful evaluation, the therapist can identify the kind of thinking, level of understanding, ability to concentrate, and capacity to work on lengthy assignments, in order to decide if verbal or nonverbal, direct or indirect, short-term or long-term treatment would be most appropriate (Ronen, 1993a).

THE INFLUENCE OF CHILDREN'S EMOTIONAL STAGE

It would be unimaginable to treat children without relating to their emotional stage as well as to their emotional needs. At different ages, children are capable of expressing different kinds of emotions. For example, preschoolers can differentiate between being "sad" and being "happy," whereas at about 10 or 11 years of age, children can differentiate between more complicated emotions such as "stressed," "depressed," and "anxious." As the ability to identify a wider variety of feelings increases, a parallel process occurs: Children grow in their capacity to differentiate between self and others, not only as separate beings, but as having different subjective ways of coping and feeling. Both of these evolving processes are necessary in order to establish and conduct meaningful relationships (Schaffer, 1996).

Emotions are elicited through the development of an attachment to significant figures. This process starts during the first few months of age, through the second year of life. At that time, specific attachment bonds become clearest, and fear begins to emerge as a dominant emotion. Those emotions include wariness of strangers and separation protests. As children grow up, during early and middle childhood, they learn to express emotion and accept emotion. By the age of 11 years and higher, children are already more likely to attribute emotional arousal to internal causes rather than to external events (Shirk & Russell, 1996; Thompson, 1989). Thus, with increasing age, children not only develop a broader range of emotional concepts, but also increasingly appreciate the psychological dimensions of emotional experience, which help them to interpret their own emotional experiences in more sophisticated ways. This new perceptiveness fosters more accurate interpretations of the direct emotional displays of others and increases children's competence at inferring emotions in others when direct cues are lacking (Thompson, 1989).

Young children are likely to rely on cognitively uncomplicated outcome-dependent emotions such as happiness or sadness, which are developed early and easily understood (e.g. "I hurt my knee, so I'm sad"). Not long afterwards, children begin mastering more complex concepts of emotion related to attributional understanding (Thompson, 1989), for instance: "I always feel sad and scared when I hurt myself, so Mom must also be feeling sad and scared right now because she hurt herself." As cognitive functions mature, new emotions emerge. Those emotions become available to the child as experiences. Then the child can comprehend differential attributions such as: "Maybe my mother feels differently from me when she gets hurt, maybe she's angry" or "Look, Mom feels sad and scared, and she didn't even hurt herself, there must be another reason." Psychologists identify cognitive–developmental transitions as preconditions for a child to be able to think about emotion (Gordon, 1989).

It is impossible to treat children without knowing at what stage of affective development the child is located. The child may be at an early developmental stage, when support and clarification of emotions are most important, or the child might already understand complex emotions such as stress, anxiety, and ambivalence, thereby indicating a readiness to accept and live with constructive criticism.

MOBILIZING THE CHILD'S MOTIVATION FOR CHANGE

Kanfer and Schefft (1988) proposed that there is no such thing as a client without motivation. Everyone is motivated. The relevant questions are: What is the person motivated towards? and How can the therapist mobilize the client's motivation toward the treatment process? A critically important and often difficult task in child psychotherapy lies in the creation and maintenance of the necessary therapeutic environment. Children come to therapy because they have been brought there: not because they have their own agenda or expected outcomes, but rather in order to comply with adults. Yet, children will not remain or invest in therapy unless they like the therapist and enjoy the therapeutic process (Ronen, 1993b, 1997b).

The quality of the relationship constitutes one of the most important features in individual child therapy (Brandell, 1992). Children will not continue treatment if they are bored, cannot easily express themselves, or if the therapist does not succeed in stimulating their curiosity, interest, motivation, and participation (Kazdin, 1988a; Ronen, 1992). The child therapist must utilize play activities, create a climate of trust, and establish a meaningful affective relationship with the child (Rose & Edelson, 1988).

The choice of techniques is also clearly intertwined with children's motivation. Technique selection should be determined by a variety of factors including the child's interests, preferences, and developmental stage, yet may be limited by the therapist's technical repertoire and propensities (Brandell, 1992; Ronen, 1992). To increase the child's enthusiastic involvement, a range of techniques such as drawing, playing, or talking may be employed.

The issue of motivation becomes more complicated when dealing with adolescents. On the one hand, youngsters at this age can concentrate longer and remain in treatment even while facing difficult turning points. They do not expect their therapist to be interesting but rather to be helpful. Therefore, they can remain in therapy if they see it as serving their own interests, such as helping them resolve a conflict with parents or teachers, or improving their social relations. On the other hand, at this stage, teenagers have other motivations. Their sensitivity to social events and social situations is already well developed (or even exaggerated). Due to their preoccupation with the peer group, as they attempt to separate from the nuclear family and to establish an individual identity, they may be more afraid of stigma or mental disorder and may feel ashamed or embarrassed, and therefore may avoid therapy.

PERSONAL STYLE, INTERESTS, AND CULTURE

Therapists need to be keenly aware of the child's personal language, thinking style, and specific interests in order to use these for communication in therapy. In addition to determining the child's extent of subjective, time-limited thinking from a cognitive standpoint as well as the child's degree of emotional comprehension and differentiation, as suggested above, this recommendation calls on the therapist to carefully tune in to the child's favorite hobbies, particular habits, interests, and specific day-to-day experiences. These will provide content areas familiar to the child that will serve as a base of reference in therapeutic communication (Ronen, 1992).

In this manner, therapists can use various tools to help maintain the child's interest and involvement. Computers can be employed for the child whose spare time is generally dedicated to this pursuit. Dancing or drama can be expedient for children who show a propensity for such artforms or who are already involved in and enjoying such extracurricular activities. Miniature cars can be used to exemplify and explain treatment goals to the child captivated by automobiles; and even television's science fiction or superhero characters and plots can provide a communicational bridge to frequent television viewers (Ronen, 1993a). These communication requirements imply that child therapists must participate actively in the child's natural environment, become familiar with the important figures in the child's life, listen to the child's predominant vocabulary and terminology, and be flexible in the use of different methods for helping the child.

An illustration of this point can be presented regarding an athletic child who excels on his varsity soccer team and spends all of his free time watching and playing sports, but who invests very little in his academic work. By focusing only on his poor academic performance, the therapist would overlook a wealth of communicational opportunities regarding the many competence areas evidenced by this child. These might include his ability to cooperate with teammates, his capacity to follow the coach's complex instructions and obey his authority, the boy's organization, planning, and perspective-taking skills, and his capacity for motivation and perseverance toward a desired goal. Recognizing that the boy has the cognitive skills and motivation to achieve success but has difficulties in generalizing these abilities to the academic domain, the therapist could introduce a variety of techniques. For example, these could encompass using sports as a metaphor, role playing, and guided imagery to identify and reinforce the child's self-esteem and train him in transferring his skills elsewhere.

While considering personal style, cultural background should be considered as well, because the meaning of children's social behavior is influenced by cultural and societal values. It is difficult to assess a child's behavior or to make decisions about his or her therapy without knowing the impact of culture on the child's and the family's behavior. Cultural factors are known to influence informal labeling as well as formal diagnostic practice. For example, Mash and Dozois (1996) proposed that shyness and oversensitivity in children have been found to be associated with peer rejection and social maladjustment in Western cultures but with leadership, school competence, and academic achievement in Chinese children in Shanghai.

* * *

In sum, the issues related to the unique nature of psychotherapy with children could easily fill an entire book in themselves. In this chapter, I have tried to emphasize some (certainly not all) of the features that need to be considered while treating children and deciding on the most appropriate techniques to help children change. In Chapter 4, I will present the way these features influence the process of decision making about assessment, treatment, evaluation, and maintenance of outcomes.

In deciding how to apply therapy with children, two major questions should be asked:

1. What are the developmental characteristics of this specific child and his/her problem (age, gender, cognitive level, emotional stage, motivation, language, thinking style, interests), and how do I believe they may affect this child's assessment, treatment design, intervention process, evaluation, and outcome maintenance?
2. What kind of technique(s) could best help me achieve my aims?

This chapter has attempted to respond to the first question, and in the next two chapters I will address the second by proposing the cognitive–constructivist and then the creative approach to serve as the clinician's techniques of choice.

2

Cognitive–Constructivist Therapy with Children

The approach to children's treatment that I propose is based on a cognitive–constructivist orientation. I will first review the basics of cognitive therapy in general and how it can be applied to the unique requirements of child therapy.

THE BASIC ASSUMPTIONS OF COGNITIVE THEORY

Cognitive therapy constitutes a holistic way of life, a way of thinking and perceiving human functioning and needs, and a way of operating within the environment in order to achieve the most effective means for accomplishing one's aims.

As a scientific approach, cognitive therapy relies on empirical studies of human behavior based on the results of behavioral assessment and constant evaluation (Hersen & Bellack, 1981). Human behavior is seen as being in a constant process of change; therefore, people are always able to render changes in their behavior. Relating to change, the same rule explaining normal human behavior can explain deviations. An important emphasis is on the interaction between behavior and environment, whereby change can be achieved by modifying either the environment or the individual.

Thinking is considered to play an important role in the etiology and maintenance of disorders (Alford & Beck, 1997; Hollon & Beck, 1994). The cognitive therapeutic approach is based on the underlying theoretical rationale that an individual's affect and behavior are largely determined by the way in which he or she structures the world (Alford & Beck, 1997; Beck, 1963, 1976; Beck et al., 1979, 1985; Mahoney, 1991). Individuals are viewed as actively involved in constructing their own reality. A person's cognitions (verbal or pictorial "events" in the stream of consciousness) are based on attitudes or assumptions (schemata) developed from previous experiences (Beck et al., 1990). Thus, all perceiving, learning, and knowing are products of an information processing system that actively selects, filters, and interprets environmental and other sensory inputs that impinge on the organism (Clark, 1995). Cognitions are considered the most important links in the chain of events leading to disordered behavior and psychological dysfunction (Powell & Oei, 1991).

As therapy is a planned, designed process, much attention has been given to the construction of the intervention process. The most familiar procedure for intervention, Gambrill's 12 steps (Gambrill et al., 1971), has provided guidelines to conduct the process of intervention. The 12 steps and their goals consist of:

1. *Inventory of problem areas.* Collects information about the whole spectrum of presented problems.
2. *Problem selection and contract.* Achieves client–therapist agreement on problem areas selected for change while stimulating client cooperation and involvement.
3. *Commitment to cooperate.* Obtains the client's agreement with the process and facilitates compliance.
4. *Specification of target behaviors.* Specifies details concerning the selected problem and demonstrates what maintains and reinforces the problem.
5. *Baseline of target behavior.* Documents pre-intervention frequency and duration of the problem, to provide a concrete foundation on which to evaluate change.
6. *Identification of problem controlling conditions.* Identifies the conditions preceding and following the problem's occurrence.
7. *Assessment of environmental resources.* Uncovers possible resources in the client's environment.
8. *Specification of behavioral objectives.* Specifies the behavioral objectives of the modification plan, and elicits the client's terminal behavioral repertoire.
9. *Formulation of a modification plan.* Selects an appropriate technique for applying the most efficient program for change.
10. *Implementation of modification plan.* Modifies behavior and focuses effort on change.
11. *Monitoring outcomes.* Collects information concerning the effectiveness of intervention.
12. *Maintenance of change.* Works to achieve maintenance and stabilization, to help prevent relapses.

Another well-accepted construction of therapy is that of Kanfer and Schefft (1988), who proposed seven treatment phases:

1. Role restructuring and creating a therapeutic alliance.
2. Developing a commitment for change.
3. Behavioral analysis.
4. Negotiating treatment objectives and methods.
5. Implementing treatment and maintaining motivation.
6. Monitoring and evaluating progress.
7. Maintenance, generalization, and termination of treatment.

THE BASICS OF CONSTRUCTIVIST THERAPY

During the last few decades, the emergence of constructivism has contributed an important new addition to cognitive therapy, emphasizing the role of emotion and therapeutic relationships in the treatment process. Many of the cognitive–behavioral therapists of today are actually cognitive–behavioral–constructivist therapists. Constructivism differs from cognitive theory in the design, assessment, evaluation, and maintenance of therapy. The goal-directed design of the treatment process that is so integral to cognitive therapy is not a crucial component in constructivist therapy. Neither is the need to continually assess and evaluate the client's progress.

Constructivism, as the latest development in cognitive theory, derives from Kelly's personal theory that views the person as a combination of scientist and architect (Kelly, 1955). According to the constructivist perspective, human beings are personal scientists who are continually creating conceptual templates from experiences (Kanfer & Schefft, 1988; Kelly, 1955; Neimeyer & Mahoney, 1995). As scientists, people organize their experiences in a way that creates meaning in their lives. Knowledge comprises the main way in which human beings regulate their perceptions of environmental events (Guidano, 1995). Knowledge about both similarities and contrasts can be elicited by the individual's continuous comparison and organization of ongoing life experiences. This knowledge is a chief component in the person's ability (as a scientist) to organize, make sense of, and give meaning to life experiences, the self, and the world. Knowledge is progressively shaped and changed in response to challenging environmental pressures (Guidano, 1995).

Viewing people as architects highlights their role in construing their own world and in constructing a personal reality, via a personal meaning making process (Kelly, 1955; Mahoney, 1991, 1995). Constructs allow humans to interpret, predict, and appropriately respond to their subsequent experiences (Neimeyer, 1995b). One's construction system varies and changes as one successively anticipates events and construes their replications. The concept of the meaning making process is based on the understanding that psychological problems are, in large part, determined by the way people construe their experiences (Kelly, 1955). The emphasis of constructivism lies on the tenet that each person is responsible for the individual way he or she organizes the way life is lived. Viewing each individual as a unique architect, the personal construct intervention advocates first attempting to understand the client and then creating an intervention appropriate for that one human being (Swell, 1995).

The way in which that particular individual understands feelings is of paramount importance according to the constructivist approach. Affect does not exist as an entity separate from cognition and vice versa (Neimeyer, 1995a; Swell, 1995). Emotions are inseparable from the cognitions that play a central role in behavior, and both constitute main components in change processes (Swell, 1995). A unique focus of constructivism lies in its emphasis on exploration, experimentation, and openness to feelings and experiences.

Neimeyer (1995c) proposed a therapeutic design based on selecting the strategic and technical preferences of constructivist therapy. He suggested strategies and techniques for six major domains of intervention:

1. *Assessment focus.* The main strategy is the exploration of personal narratives, and the preferred intervention techniques comprise identification of central metaphors, life review, and laddering techniques.
2. *Goal of therapy.* The strategy is creative rather than corrective, and the following techniques are used: stream of consciousness, exploration, and reprocessing of emotions.
3. *Interpretation of emotion.* The strategic treatment of negative emotions is integral to constructive change, and the intervention techniques include reprocessing of emotional schemata.
4. *Level of intervention.* The strategy is attention to selfhood processes, and the intervention incorporates the enactment of deep role relationships.
5. *Style of therapy.* Using a personal rather than authoritative strategy, the intervention style adopts a "not knowing" approach and utilizes elaboration of metaphors or stories.
6. *Approach to resistance.* Resistance in therapy is strategically understood as a legitimate attempt to protect core-ordering processes, and intervention techniques promote the allowance of resistance and externalization of problems.

THE COGNITIVE–CONSTRUCTIVIST VIEW OF THERAPY

Cognitive–constructivist therapy is based on working toward an understanding of the client and then intervening in how that client anticipates experiences

(Swell, 1995) by creating an intervention appropriate for that one human being. Therapy focuses on the *person*, rather than on the pathological response, and its main purpose is to help people cope better with their lives. This therapeutic approach comprises a very careful, continuous assessment process that attempts to analyze the particular client's needs, our knowledge about the specific problem, and the client's skills and abilities, in order to determine the treatment of choice. The same problem could be treated differently as a result of decision making related to personal, environmental, and behavioral considerations. Intervention methods vary and can include verbal as well as experiential techniques.

Primary emphasis in cognitive therapy is placed on cognitive processes, including the identification and modification of individuals' core beliefs, conditional assumptions, and automatic thoughts. One basic tenet in cognitive–constructivist therapy is that the manner in which individuals process information influences their emotions, behavior, and physiology in reliable, predictable ways. Another is that human problems derive from irrational thinking (Beck et al., 1979). In order to address these difficulties, cognitive–constructivist therapy aims to raise awareness of and modify cognitive processes such as perceptions, self-statements, attributions, expectations, and problem solving skills. In addition, therapy is targeted toward helping people in identifying their distorted automatic thoughts; understanding the way those thoughts elicit emotions; and viewing behavior as the outcome of a process combining thoughts and emotions (Alford & Beck, 1997; Beck et al., 1979).

Change processes in therapy derive from attempts to convert irrational, automatic, or maladaptive emergent core schemata into more rational, mediated, or adaptive beliefs and thought processes. During treatment, changes are regulated and modeled step by step, and maintenance processes are aimed at preserving the functional continuity and sense of oneness inherent in selfhood structures (Guidano, 1995). Human change processes are characterized by an oscillating and uncertain pattern, both in their path and in their timing from one step to the next (Mahoney, 1991).

Rosenbaum and Ronen (1998) summarized the seven basic features of cognitive–constructivist therapy (and therapeutic supervision). The first comprises meaning making processes. The goal of therapy is to help clients develop a new and more suitable way of understanding and accepting the way they behave. The intervention process, therefore, is directed toward understanding the meanings that the particular client attributes to his or her life, or the meanings attributed to specific events in the person's life.

The second component consists of systematic and goal-directed processes. Treatment is planned and executed, and the therapeutic hour is constructed (Beck, 1976), with an emphasis on the need to define problems, goals, expectations, means to achieve these goals, assessment, and evaluation of the process.

The third component involves practicing and experiencing. Cognitive (and constructivist) therapy is not a talking therapy but rather a doing therapy that encompasses practicing and experiencing as central components. Interventions vary and can be verbal or nonverbal, using experiential methods such as role assignments, imagery training, metaphors, writing methods, etc. (Mahoney, 1991).

The fourth consists of collaborative effort. Therapist and client are expected to enter into an alliance and to collaborate on joint work in order to achieve the goals of therapy.

The fifth component constitutes client-focused intervention. Cognitive–constructivist intervention should aim at treating the person, rather than treating the problem. This view focuses on the person as a whole, and concentrates on the client's feelings, thoughts, and way of living, not only on the client's problem.

The sixth component comprises facilitating change processes. This component emphasizes the important role of the therapist in pursuing effective strategies and techniques to help the client change (Rosenbaum & Ronen, 1998).

The seventh component concerns empowerment and resourcefulness. All of the previous features are actually aimed at empowering clients by training them in self-control skills for self-help and independent functioning.

These seven features emphasize the role of practicing and experiencing in cognitive behavior, both in the therapeutic setting (in the form of rehearsing skills) and in the natural environment (as homework assignments).

CHILD DEVELOPMENT IN VIEW OF COGNITIVE–CONSTRUCTIVIST THEORIES

The first chapter in this book focused on viewing children as undergoing a constant process of change or, in other words, a "form of motion." Cognitive–constructivist therapy with children, therefore, focuses on the way one constructs one's perceptions as well as one's motion through development. Development is seen as a branching network of experiments designed to get to know the world, with complexity increasing in both depth (how much do I know about X?) and breadth (how many Xs do I know about? What do they have to do with each other?). Very small children do not have verbal labels to distinguish between the above, but they do have preverbal constructs that they use for different distinctions with which to predict their experiences. Young children may be limited in their verbal abilities and may lack the cognitive skills necessary to explain their emotions and behaviors. However, they do feel, understand, and behave in specific ways that stem from their experiences. Primarily, a child's construct system develops structurally over time, as the child increases his or her degree of organization.

The development of the self is an active learning process stemming from a specific set of evolutionary constraints. The study of child development originates in infants' learning. Children become progressively able to recognize, define, and evaluate others and, through these processes, themselves. This learning is acquired via their interactions with their environment. In particular, attachment in human functioning plays an important role in children's learning. In his attachment theory, Bowlby (1969, 1973, 1988) described the main factors that contribute to the structuring of self-knowledge. These developmental stages can be considered as a progressive series of transformations, beginning with the basic self-organization and ending with the emergence of a conscious self-image and a structured self-identity:

Preschool years (ages 3–5). Organization of basic deep structural relations occurs, affording relatively stable patterns of self and world perceptions.

Childhood or primary school age (ages 6–11; associated with Piaget's (1924) stage of concrete operations). Qualitative changes transpire, permitting differentiated organization of experiences.

Adolescence and youth (12–18 years; Piaget's formal operations stage). Qualitative changes in knowing allow the individual to experience the self both as an already existing agent and as something to be discovered through a process of self-reflection.

Adulthood. Adulthood begins as the self emerges as "a knower," with an understanding of the full sense of personal identity and an active role in one's own continuing self-organization.

ADAPTING COGNITIVE–CONSTRUCTIVIST PSYCHOTHERAPY TO CHILDREN

Constructivist therapy with children is quite a new area. Therefore, most of the material mentioned in this chapter is mainly cognitive grounded. Cognitive therapy is implemented with children on the basis of the assumption that their deviant behavior reflects deficiencies in particular processes or an inability to use or to apply certain cognitive skills (Kendall & Braswell, 1985). Examples may be an impulsive cognitive style, deficits in taking the perspective of others, or misattributions of others' intentions (Kazdin, 1988a). Cognitive therapy with children aims to help them select appropriate behaviors for everyday life, focusing on the process rather than on the outcome; teaching the child to engage in a step-by-step approach for solving problems; and combining behavioral, cognitive, and constructivist methods to lead the child to effective solutions (Kazdin, 1988a).

As applications of cognitive therapy with children have progressed, the field has developed differently from cognitive treatments of adults. Therapy with children has not been based on a unified theoretical model that would assess and address childhood disorders as well as provide a framework for evaluating the proposed techniques (Ronen, 1995, 1997b). Instead, cognitive therapy has become an umbrella term for different treatment techniques that can be offered in many different sequences and permutations. Most of the cognitive work being utilized with children either addresses one specific problem, or one specific technique. The specific problems targeted may include fear of going out at night, thinking before starting a test, improving reading skills, etc. (see Copeland, 1982; Kanfer et al., 1975; Kendall & Braswell, 1985). The specific techniques that have been addressed include, for example, instruction in the use of cognitive mediational strategies to guide children's behavior and thus improve their adjustment (e.g. self-talk or self-recording; Durlak et al., 1991). Cognitive therapy applications, thus far, have not adequately converged to provide a comprehensive compilation of assessment and treatment techniques to deal with the multiple aspects and components of prevalent childhood disorders such as attention-deficit/hyperactivity or anxiety disorders.

As described above, cognitive–constructivist treatments emphasize the link between the person and the social environment, viewing the environment as strongly influencing behavior, emotions, and thoughts as well as the reverse. Cognitive therapy with children and families in particular underscores situational influences on behavior (Mash & Dozois, 1996; Mash & Terdal, 1988). Whenever a child is concerned, the family is involved; and most treatment settings include the child within his or her family. The therapy is system-oriented, describing and understanding the characteristics of the child and the family, the context in which such characteristics are manifested, and the structural organizations and functional relationships that exist between situations and behaviors, thoughts, and emotions (Mash & Terdal, 1988).

Children's constructions of their own reality, like older people's, is more important than so-called "objective" events (Mahoney, 1991). This possible incongruity highlights the important issue of how people's lives should be understood and lived (Rychlak, 1968). It is necessary to underscore the importance of subjective reports by the children themselves regarding their own levels of distress and other emotional reactions, for the purposes of assessment and intervention. As described in Chapter 1, research relating to different sources of evaluation has demonstrated discrepancies in the way parents, children, and teachers perceive, experience, or evaluate situations (Ronen, 1997b; Rosenbaum & Ronen, 1997).

Cognitive therapy has been considered a promising treatment strategy for a wide range of children's problems (Dush et al., 1989; Gresham, 1981), as long as the therapist is able to adapt techniques to the children's developmental needs (Ronen, 1992, 1997b). Adapting cognitive–constructivist techniques to children depends, to a large extent, on the therapist's ability to translate cognitive–constructivist concepts and techniques in a way that is clear, understandable, and sensible to children and their parents (Knell, 1993; Ronen, 1992, 1993b). Treating children requires an adaptation of the basic cognitive–constructivist model to include assessment of developmental factors such as age, gender, cognitive level, and the kind of problems referred, which can contribute to the selection of the most suitable treatment mode (Ronen, 1993b).

The treatment of children, even at a very young age, may be facilitated by an approach relating to the "inner," subjective point of view, that is, focusing on one's personal meaning making process and the constructs of one's experiences. This contrasts with an approach looking at the "outside" reality comprised by objective experiences or by adult perceptions of children's experiences, which often mistakenly tend to be regarded as the primary criterion for mediating the child's behavior. Relating to their inner world is essential before trying to incur a shift in the meaning children attribute to an event. As underscored by cognitive and constructivist therapists, the child's goal should consist of finding a new meaning or inventing a new interpretive framework for the world (Mahoney, 1991), rather than fighting the old meaning. The child's therapist must try to reach a workable understanding of what the event means for the child (Shirk & Russell, 1996). Therapists must (within their own conceptual system), learn to feel what the specific child feels. They should know how he or she perceives the event, what the child believes this reaction stands for, and how the child has constructed his or her own reality in a manner that might be devastating in the long run. What makes the child look at it the way he or she does? How will this view affect the child's present or future functioning? What should be done in order to help the child reconstruct the event into another frame of reference?

Great emphasis must be placed on the importance of the therapeutic relationship for the child's process of change. Safran and Segal (1990) stressed the significance of the therapeutic alliance and relationship in order to develop an ability for change. With children, again, this point cannot be underscored enough. It has been suggested that a child will not continue therapy or perform the homework assignments or take part in the role plays and exercises, unless he or she cares for and trusts the therapist and feels safe within the relationship (Ronen, 1993a).

Treating children is a challenge that cannot be optimally met unless the therapist can accept the child, the unique features of child development and childhood disorders, and the specific child's language and way of thinking. The therapist must then combine all these with cognitive theory in order to fulfill the main aim of intervention: helping children to help themselves. The goal of therapy, therefore, is not to impose verbiage where once was emotion but to build structure where once was anxiety, generating courage for experimentation.

BASIC PRINCIPLES IN APPLYING COGNITIVE–CONSTRUCTIVIST THERAPY WITH CHILDREN

In line with the review of cognitive and constructivist therapies and their application to children presented in this chapter, several basic principles should direct the cognitive–constructivist therapist in his or her work:

1. Children are always able to change themselves.

2. However young they may be, children have the ability to learn, and it is the therapist's responsibility to find the best way to foster that learning.
3. Concepts in therapy must be adapted to the child's age, stage, and language.
4. Children's behavior is strongly linked with their environment, and therapy must relate to both.
5. The links between the child's thoughts, emotions, and behaviors must be of central focus, along with the idea that a change in one realm is followed by a change in the others.
6. The child, rather than the pathological problem, should be treated.

Kanfer and Schefft (1988) proposed six thinking rules to direct the therapist in conducting treatment:

1. *Think behavior.* Often, therapists think problems. They concentrate on the client's problem, making assumptions and interpretations regarding its causes. Action should be the main dimension on which interchanges in therapy are focused.
2. *Think solution.* Most often therapists devote more time to thinking of difficulties and problems than to finding solutions. A full problem description requires knowledge not only of the current situation or state but also of a more desirable future, and some indication of how to achieve it.
3. *Think positive.* Just as therapists help the client to think positively and to focus on small changes and positive forces rather than on difficulties, they must themselves also aspire to positive thinking and reinforce positive outcomes.
4. *Think small steps.* Although clients are usually interested in the major, significant changes in their lives, rapid and extreme changes are difficult to obtain. Targeting small gradual changes reduces fears, motivates clients, and helps therapists observe and pinpoint difficulties. An accumulation of many small changes constitutes one final, large, and significant change.
5. *Think flexible.* This rule challenges therapists to be creative, modify their traditional interventions, and try to adapt themselves to clients' needs. Gambrill (1990) suggested that therapists look for disconfirming evidence that points to alternatives. They should try to understand other people's points of view (instead of being convinced by their own point of view), use language carefully, watch out for vivid data, move beyond the illusion of understanding, complement clear thinking skills with knowledge, and ask about accuracy.
6. *Think future.* Many therapeutic approaches focus on the past and its role on the client's present. Cognitive therapy challenges therapists to think

toward the future, predicting how their client will cope and how they themselves would like to be different or better in the future.

As can be seen in this chapter, cognitive–constructivist therapy is based on behavior, cognitions, and emotions. This seems to be complicated. However, it can be successfully applied to children if the therapist takes into account the nature of childhood and can translate the cognitive objectives into suitable concepts the child can understand and benefit from. Chapter 5 will describe in detail an intervention model based on cognitive–constructivist theories and applied to children.

3

Creative Intervention

Applying cognitive–constructivist therapy with children accentuates the need to facilitate development, empowering children and using their positive ability for change. This is achieved not only through verbal therapy but also through metaphors, imagination, role-playing, and a range of other creative means. The creative responsibility for change is shared between the therapist, who proposes new experiences, and the child, who needs to try them.

Creative therapy, for me, is not a self-contained theory, nor is it a structured mode of intervention. Creative therapy as advanced in this book constitutes a way of thinking. It mobilizes the therapist's flexibility to adapt, invent, or adjust techniques until the best means is discovered to help a specific child change. It also offers a way to learn about and identify the unique nature of each child. The individual's characteristics, interests, hobbies, and natural skills can be identified for use in therapy to facilitate the child's learning and to foster his or her expression of diverse thoughts and emotions in the manner best suited to that nature. Creative therapy, therefore, is the optimal route for adapting cognitive–constructivist therapy to children's developmental and individual needs.

DEFINING CREATIVITY

Creativity is constructing and appreciating crafted transformations, in other words, a living out of the transformational imperative in human beings to create something new (Feldman, 1988). The primary criterion for calling a given product creative is that it is to be novel, at least for the individual producing it. Sometimes, this implies a major departure from what was known at that time (Weisberg, 1993). However, it is not enough for the product to be novel; it should be of value, or be appropriate to the cognitive demands of the situation. Moreover, transformational creativity does not have to be evidenced by an artistic product.

Rather, evidence for its presence can be found in the processes of self-creation, an applied creativity that tackles the never-ceasing negotiations of life: family, friends, associates, career, personal style, inner experiences, and general behavior (Carlsen, 1995).

Csikszentmihalyi (1966) proposed a provocative reconceptualization of the concept of creativity, emphasizing the role of societal judgment of value. His theory presented a cyclical process: An individual produces some new work; however, in order for that work to be considered as creative, it must be examined by others and be accepted as of value. Therefore, creativity is not only a matter of being novel, or of cognitive importance, but also of socially recognized value.

Creativity can be an openness to new ways of seeing. It can also be an intuition, an alertness to opportunity, a liking for complexity, or a challenge to find simplicity. It might reflect an independence of judgment that questions assumptions, a willingness to take risks, or an unconventionality of thought that allows odd connections to be made (Carlsen, 1995). Weisberg (1993) explained creativity as a process of logical thinking that uses rules of inference to produce new knowledge. Each thinking rule is dependent upon the other and facilitates the new ideas as an outcome of what we already know.

THE CREATIVE PROCESS

There have been many attempts to understand the creative process. In the past, creativity was viewed as a matter of genius, pointing to creative achievements as the result of extraordinary individuals employing extraordinary thought processes (Weisberg, 1993). This view explains the origin and development of creative works by postulating special thinking processes that allow individuals to break away from the habitual and the ordinary, in what is often called "breaking the set." This view focuses on the different levels of thinking, sensitivity, and mental processes of creative people. There have been three assumptions behind the search for psychological characteristics that underlie creative genius. The first assumption is that genius is a measurable psychological characteristic or trait. Second, any personal characteristics unique to creative individuals, whatever they turn out to be, are causally related to creativity. The third is that the quality of "possessing genius" is assumed to be a permanent, or at least a relatively permanent characteristic of the individual (Weisberg, 1993).

There are some unique individuals (e.g. Einstein, Picasso, Freud, etc.) who are recognized as an inspiration and an influence on the entire world; however, most of us do not produce creative inventions that change the planet. The issue of individual differences points to the fact that all creative processes are not of the same degree of importance (Weisberg, 1993), suggesting that the genius view of creativity is a myth.

Accepting the fact that creativity can be learned and acquired by a wide range of people has led to the questions: How is a creative work produced? and What are the psychological characteristics of creative people? Human beings can perform many sorts of activities creatively, ranging from painting to cooking to studying the origin of the universe. A set of skills, talents, and motivations seems necessary, but, most of all, years of work and persistence activate creativity. In fact, underlying some of the most extraordinary inventions we can find ordinary thought processes, the ability to conduct lengthy laboratory studies, and the capacity to accept feedback and be consistent.

CHARACTERISTICS OF CREATIVE PEOPLE

Many researchers have tried to describe the essence of creative people. Barron (1988) viewed the creative person as someone who challenges assumptions. Someone who dares to question what most people accept as truth. Who recognizes and creates new patterns, sees new paths, and makes new and unusual connections in bringing together ideas. This person takes risks and produces daring new ideas; seizes the chance to take advantage of the unexpected; and constructs networks to form associations between people for an exchange of ideas. Such a process-based definition suggests the uniquely human capacity to transform the bits and pieces of experience into new patterns of significance and personal understanding. This capacity enables the person to go beyond solutions, to transcend convention, to step into the uncharted territories of innovative thoughts and ideas, and be open to the here-and-now (Carlsen, 1995).

May's (1975) work adds some personality features to the composite of creative persons. The addition is the view of creative people as having the courage to create, as possessing the wisdom and integrity that triumphs over ignorance and despair, and as demonstrating a caring for the generations, their culture, and their world that helps them overcome narcissistic preoccupations. In addition, Hurwich (1992) and LeClerc (1992) studied characteristics of older creative people and found they were able to experience life as meaningful, hold optimistic perceptions of health, maintain close relationships, continue to grow, live in the present, and practice spiritual development.

Csikszentmihalyi (1966) claimed that, in order to be creative, a person must internalize the entire system that makes creativity possible. Therefore, creative people are remarkable in their ability to adapt to almost any situation and to make do with whatever is at hand to reach their goals. He viewed creative people as characterized by paradoxical attributes, along the lines of the following ten paradoxical dimensions:

1. They have a great deal of physical energy but at the same time can be quiet and rest.

2. They tend to be smart, yet also naive.
3. They can combine playfulness and discipline.
4. They alternate between imagination and fantasy on the one hand, and a rooted sense of reality on the other.
5. They harbor opposite tendencies on the continuum between extroversion and introversion.
6. They are remarkably humble and proud at the same time.
7. They can escape the rigid dichotomy of what is a masculine or a feminine behavior.
8. They are thought to be rebellious and independent.
9. Often they are passionate about their work, yet they can be objective about it as well.
10. They are open and sensitive, which exposes them to suffering and pain yet also to a great deal of enjoyment.

ART AS A CREATIVE INTERVENTION

Life does imitate art, as evidenced by how we change in response to images. One of the most well known creative modes of psychotherapy is art therapy, which takes us into the primary sources of sacred and psychological experience if we allow the shamans and spirits to emerge once again from images and imaginations (McNiff, 1992). McNiff described art therapy as a therapy of soul, which extends to every life situation. He proposed that embracing the soul's debased expression as expressed in the images of art and dreams involves a shift in consciousness that transforms psychotherapeutic values.

Every art form is a dramatic enactment. Stories are constantly being told, bodies are always in motion. Experience with art materials helps us to see how the flourishing imagination embraces diverse faculties. We learn to follow expression in its varied movements. In art therapy, the environment of the room is transformed as people begin to interact creatively with their pictures. When this shift occurs, the tone of feeling immediately changes, imagination enters the room, and an unconscious sense of sacred spectacle, affect, and support from others is established (McNiff, 1992). Like others, McNiff believes that creativity necessitates risks. "Nothing will happen unless a person begins and risks failures, and there will be constant failures and restarts and changes of directions along the way, all of which are essential to the emergence of something fresh and surprising" (p. 34).

CREATIVE PSYCHOTHERAPISTS

Carlsen (1995) has proposed that a creative therapist is one who is called on to compare and contrast the differing ways that a client can make the world cohere, rather than one who avoids this demand. The task is to help clients bring order out of personal chaos, that is, to help them transform personal confusion and pain into a more meaningful, fulfilling program of life.

Mahoney (1991) described the creative psychotherapist as one who helps the client explore and experience himself or herself and the world in different ways. These new ways challenge ordinary, familiar patterns and consolidate embodiment, emotion, feeling, sensing, and thinking into one entity.

A creative psychotherapist is one who can adapt the treatment process to the client's unique and individual needs, using the modes, strategies, and techniques that can best suit the client's way of thinking or designing a new intervention from which the client can learn and benefit the most.

TECHNIQUES TO FACILITATE CREATIVITY

Many methods of teaching creativity have been developed over the years. Creative thought is assumed to involve attacking a problem from a new direction, which implies flexibility of thought. Therefore, an important step toward creativity is the phase of brainstorming, which includes ruling out criticism, welcoming the freewheeling, wanting quantity, and improving and complementing suggestions (Weisberg, 1993). Weisberg presented a table of methods for increasing creativity such as list making, questioning assumptions, attribute listing, analogies, incubation, and problem solving. Other guides for creativity include skills such as breaking out of old patterns or ways of thinking, keeping options open, suspending judgment, thinking broadly, breaking out of scripts, taking fresh perspectives, and using tricks.

In light of his ten characteristics of creative people, Csikszentmihalyi (1966) proposed that training in the excessive investment of attention into selfish goals could enhance personal creativity and energy. First, no one can be creative while suffering from hunger, cold, or pain. Second, one needs to wake up every morning with a specific goal to look forward to. If people do things right, these goals can become enjoyable. Habits, a fixed schedule, and discipline should thus protect creativity. Csikszentmihalyi emphasized, for example, the importance of trying to be surprised by something every day, as well as trying to surprise at least one other person daily, and he suggested keeping a daily record of these surprises. He also focused on the importance of "flow." Another suggestion was to look for personality traits and try to shift between paradoxical ones, such as openness and closedness.

Creativity in this book relates both to the therapist and the child. The therapist is being asked to be attentive to the child, to be creative, to be flexible in his or her way of thinking, and to elicit different ways for facilitating the child's change process. The child is being asked to be creative in letting himself or herself use different modes, skills, and techniques such as play, paint, sculpture, imagery, etc., and in mobilizing all these in order to learn and change.

It is beyond the scope of this book to describe in detail all of the possible means for improving creativity. However, I do hope I was able at least to present the flavor and significance of creativity and the creative process as an important and integral part of therapy. The case studies presented in Part III of the book illustrate the way creative thinking can be incorporated into children's cognitive therapy to design the most effective intervention for change.

II

Applying an Intervention Model

The first part of this book (Chapters 1–3) presented a basic review of children's unique characteristics as they affect child therapy, an examination of cognitive–constructivist therapy as modified to suit children, and a general view of creative intervention.

In the second part of the book (Chapters 4 and 5), I will show how I have consolidated these three components into one concise approach to guide the decision making and intervention process in cognitive–constructivist therapy with children. Chapter 4 proposes guidelines for decision making, which steer the therapist through a set of questions such as whether a child needs therapy, which setting is best, and what kind of techniques should be applied. Then, in Chapter 5, a self-control intervention model is described, emphasizing the "how to do what" of children's treatment.

4

Making Decisions on Therapy

Cognitive–constructivist theory and therapy, and particularly the self-control model that I will present in Chapter 5, constitute the *content* of my basic intervention approach, encompassing my way of thinking, analyzing, and working creatively toward change. Yet, the unique characteristics of childhood and developmental considerations have a central impact on the *process* of my therapeutic decision making. Particularly, the referred problem's characteristics; a range of developmental issues; child, therapist, and family variables; and individual differences are all aspects that are integrated into the following guidelines for the creative therapist.

Kanfer and Schefft (1988) proposed that clinical change is only one part in the sequence that leads from first awareness of a problem to its resolution. In the case of children, this process includes both the environment and the child. The process relates both to the ability of the environment (parents, teachers, peers) and/or the child himself or herself to acknowledge the problem's existence. Also, both the environment and the child need to define and evaluate it in order to decide that the problem will not resolve itself spontaneously and that treatment is necessary.

A PREFACE: ASSESSMENT AS AN ESSENTIAL TREATMENT FEATURE FROM START TO FINISH

Traditional views of treatment separate the diagnostic component from the treatment component, emphasizing the former as a preliminary phase of treatment. In this book, I would like to present another, more integrative view, which upholds that diagnosis and assessment are not limited to certain early stages but rather must encompass integral parts of the entire therapeutic proceedings. Assessment may be viewed as a nonstop process of decision making by the therapist during child intervention. It comprises a constant process of asking questions and conducting continual assessment, which begins at the time of the referral, continues throughout intervention, and culminates when treatment outcomes are evaluated and maintained. In each phase of intervention, the assessment and questioning processes differ in their emphasis or focus, yet they must always be asked in relation to the specific problem in that specific child at his/her specific age.

Assessment as proposed here may be differentiated from the work of diagnosis. Assessment comprises a dynamic process of checking and rechecking information, asking questions about hypotheses and assumptions, and looking for change in the child's functioning. Assessment usually constitutes an analysis of the therapist's impressions and reports from the client's environment. Diagnosis constitutes the strict comparison of the child's behavior to clinical criteria reflecting standardized norms. For the purpose of diagnosis, therapists often use valid and reliable assessment tools such as tests, questionnaires, and clinical diagnostic criteria. During the ongoing process of assessment that is part and parcel of child intervention, some phases require that the therapist use diagnostic procedures. For example, at the beginning of therapy, a need arises to arrive at a specific diagnosis, for the purpose of making a decision about the need to treat the child and determining the setting, etc. Another phase calling for diagnostic evaluation may occur at the termination of therapy, when it is necessary to use diagnostic procedures to evaluate treatment outcomes. Evaluative assessment at the end of therapy compares the child's current behavior to baseline levels, in order to learn about the efficacy of the treatment and the extent of change exhibited by the client. Often, assessment is conducted to reexamine the initial diagnosis and to decide whether or not it is still appropriate.

In the cognitive–constructivist approach, assessment begins with the therapist's initial meeting with the child and parents but continues throughout the intervention, until the termination of treatment. Therefore, I will not relate to assessment as a separate stage of intervention, but rather will incorporate it into the various phases, emphasizing times when stricter use of assessment measures should be implemented for purposes of diagnosis and evaluation.

In Chapter 2, I presented proposals of how therapy should be designed. In light of cognitive therapy the most familiar procedure for intervention is Gambrill's 12 steps (Gambrill et al., 1971) that provide guidelines to conduct the process of intervention. This procedure comprises 12 goal-directed, structured, gradual steps (Gambrill et al., 1971; Kanfer & Schefft, 1988). Constructivist psychotherapy, on the other hand, is not as structured as the cognitive one. Intervention is also a planned process, but more flexible, more apt to the client's specific needs at that specific moment. Neimeyer (1995c) has proposed construction of the therapeutic process based on selecting the main strategic and technical preferences of constructivist therapy, relating to six major domains of intervention (see Chapter 3).

In this chapter, I will propose guidelines for designing therapy in line with a cognitive–constructivist orientation based on children's specific needs. These guidelines provide a sequence of questions reflecting the major decisions encountered by the child psychotherapist and describing the relevant assessment methods for each phase: *Does this child need therapy or not?* (Phase 1), *How can this child's referral and goals for change be classified?* (Phase 2), *What is the right setting for treatment?* (Phase 3), *What are the optimal modes and techniques for intervention?* (Phase 4), and *What outcome was achieved by treatment and how can it be maintained?* (Phase 5).

PHASE 1: HOW TO DECIDE IF THERAPY IS NEEDED BASED ON THE UNIQUE NATURE OF CHILDHOOD

The first chapter of this book elaborated on the unique nature of child psychotherapy in light of children's rapid changes, the normal basis of childhood disorders, the discrepancies between chronological, emotional, and cognitive stages, gender differences, children's motivations, and so on. I propose that all of these unique characteristics of children should comprise important features in the process of decision making with regard to whether a given referred child should be treated or not.

Wozner (1985) proposed a procedure for making a decision as to when a problem should be regarded as sufficient for beginning intervention. He highlighted three main issues to be appraised: the probability of the treatment's success, the difficulties expected in resolving the presented problem, and the severity of the problem. Wozner claimed that the best conditions for intervention are afforded by the selection of a behavior problem that: (a) has a good prognosis, that is, good chances for success; (b) is not difficult to change; (c) has goals that can be achieved in a short time; and (d) does not require urgent intervention. Unfortunately, we are often involved with cases where a problem is severe and urgent, motivation is low, and the prognosis is not good. Therefore, only a combination of features can help in making a decision as to whether such a problem should be treated or not.

From my experience, when a child is capable of creating a good alliance with the therapist, even severe problems with low known success rates can be treated and then changed. On the other hand, psychotherapists should not overlook the negative impact of entering therapy for some families. Therapists are immersed in the world of mental health, show a clear proclivity toward self-disclosure, and accept the idea of receiving help for problems (Schaffer, 1990). Thus, they may not always give full consideration to families' concerns about stigma, fears of therapy, and the concurrent effects on self-esteem (Ronen, 1997a,b). Clinicians certainly must address these emotional responses at the onset of establishing a therapeutic relationship (Shirk & Russell, 1996). Moreover, if only a mild gain is expected as a result of therapy, or if the anticipated rate of spontaneous recovery is high, it is in the prospective clients' best interests that we therapists should learn to turn them away. Clinicians should not underestimate the motivating effect for the child and family's subsequent efforts to cope with the referred problems, in the event that they are assessed by a professional and told that they do not need treatment (Ronen, 1997a).

The first phase in any intervention process necessarily entails making a decision as to whether or not the referred child's presented problem actually necessitates intervention. This phase calls for the consideration of a blend of assessment and diagnostic criteria. Four main sets of variables can guide this decision: problem variables, environmental variables, child and family variables, and treatment variables (Ronen, 1997b). Each of the four variables combines a set of questions that the therapist should ask and important features to be looked for, in order to decide whether or not the presented problem necessitates professional intervention. Table 4.1 outlines the components of each of the four variables in this first phase of the intervention process, as well as the assessment tools and the main sources that can help answer these questions. More detailed guidelines follow the table.

As can be seen in Table 4.1, the described components can illuminate the child's present state, the past history of the disorder, and/or future expectations. The decision about the need for therapy is an outcome of examining the past progression of the disorder, the child's current state, the prognosis, and strengths that will help in rendering future changes.

Problem Variables

The first aspect of assessment relates to the nature of the problem. When a child is referred, the therapist should first ask: Is the problem known, and does it fit any of the diagnostic criteria? As a general rule, a problem should be treated if it fits recognized clinical diagnostic criteria (e.g. the *Diagnostic and Statistical Manual of Mental Disorders – DSM-IV –* of the American Psychiatric Association, 1994). However, often a problem does not fulfill the criteria for clinical diagnosis but nevertheless disturbs the child and family (Mash & Dozois, 1996).

Thus, the second question regarding the problem's characteristics concerns its frequency and severity. If its frequency is increasing (or at times, remaining stable), especially if it poses a risk to the child's future (see below), therapy should be initiated. In contrast, if the problem is improving (or perhaps stabilized), it might be worthwhile to wait and see if it will improve spontaneously. Careful collection

Table 4.1. Phase 1: Does the Child Need Therapy or Not?

Variable	Questions to be asked	Time period	Assessment & diagnostic tools	Main sources of information
Problem	1. Diagnostic criteria?	Past	Intake interview & clinical diagnostic criteria (*DSM-IV*)	Parents, impressions from: child, parents, teachers
	2. Frequency of the disorder?	Present	Reports from environment	Teachers, parents
	3. Risk for the child's future?	Future	Direct observation, child testing	Child
Developmental and environmental	1. Disorder's resemblance to other children in the same environment? 2. Disorder's resemblance to the child's age group? 3. Disorder's resemblance to the child's sex group? 4. Family's view of the problem as severe, necessitating intervention?	Present	Diagnostic criteria, family interview	Reference materials, literature, family interview, teacher interview
Child & family	1. Child's motivation for change? 2. Family's motivation for change? 3. Kind of existing support systems? 4. Child's emotional state and how it's affected by the problem?	Present	Interview with the child and the family	Family interview, report from previous therapists
Treatment	1. Available prognosis? 2. Probability of spontaneous recovery? 3. Likelihood of therapy rendering a change? 4. Changes in the child's life following therapy? 5. Chances of developing a good therapeutic relationship?	Future	Diagnostic criteria, impressions from session with the child	Reference materials, literature, therapist, child

of historical data on the referred problem's frequency and stability and use of diagnostic references will provide the information necessary to determine if treatment is indicated.

A third step in problem-related decision making is determining if the referred problem poses a risk to the child's future. Here therapy may be warranted even if the problem has improved, when it appears that the problem might pose a risk to the child's well being in the present or the future (Ronen, 1998a). For example, a 6-year-old boy who was about to enter school suffered from encopresis. Over the past 2 years, the soiling behavior had improved. He no longer restrained for more than 2 days, instead of his previous week long retentions, and he now soiled his pants only 2–3 times weekly instead of daily. However, the fact that he was starting a new school posed a social risk; peers could reject him because of his soiling behavior, thus pointing to the need to treat him although he had already improved remarkably. Often, we intervene with children to prevent the problem from growing (in secondary or tertiary prevention), to prevent future danger, and to avoid future risk. This first set of questions regarding the problem itself in effect encompasses the clinical diagnosis of the behavior.

Developmental and Environmental Variables

It is impossible to decide whether or not a child needs therapy without comparing the presented problem to the second set of variables: the child's age and sex group, and social norms. The questions to be asked here concern the problem's coincidence with that of other children in this child's environment, its prevalence among the child's age and sex group, and the family's view of the problem's severity (Mash & Terdal, 1988; Ronen, 1993c). An indication for treatment is when the problem does deviate from the child's age and sex group, and from environmental norms (e.g. a 12-year-old boy who is afraid of the dark while most children of his age have already overcome this fear). In contrast, sometimes the occurrence of a disorder might result from social norms or role modeling, and does not appear deviant while looking at the child's own social and cultural environment. It is then important to ask whether or not there is risk to the child's well-being (e.g. a child who still wets the bed at the age of 3 years or who has not begun to talk at the age of 2). Under such conditions, therapy is generally contraindicated. These questions provide a diagnosis based on developmental rather than clinical criteria.

Child and Family Variables

The third consideration in deciding whether or not to initiate treatment relates to child and family variables, which are of the utmost importance for the success of intervention. First and foremost, does the child have motivation for change? Therapists must take into account that children's motivational status is not a given, as they are almost always referred by adults. Motivational attitudes among the child as well as the family are of great consequence for decision making, considering their influence on the child's cooperation and collaboration with treatment assignments. For example, even when a problem is extremely severe and its prognosis is very poor, strong motivation for change might color the whole situation differently (Kanfer & Schefft, 1988). Another example would be when a problem is common in the child's environment, posing a low future risk, as described above, yet the child views the problem as deviant or it disturbs the family. In such a case, treatment can still be applied, even when the problem does not meet the above criteria regarding its nature and its developmental and environmental features. Conversely, when child or family motivation is lacking in a case with high future risk, the first step of therapy will be to identify any area of motivation in the clients and use it to increase motivation for change.

The third question to be asked in this set of variables consists of: Is there social and family support for change? Once again, as problematic as the situation may be, peer and family support might energize the child for change. Support systems can render an impact on a child's condition and are therefore crucial for treatment. For example, an 11-year-old girl with cancer underwent surgical procedures and all the difficulties of treatment while her friends kept visiting her, sending her letters, calling her, and updating her on everything going on in school and with friends. This social support strengthened her inner resources to cope with the difficult process she was undergoing. This question focuses on an assessment of the child's cultural and environmental support.

The fourth question in this set of variables consists of the impact of the child's emotional state on decision making. For example, a child may be severely distressed by seemingly innocuous incidents or problems (e.g. a teacher's scolding, a one-time occurrence of soiling at kindergarten, or very mild stuttering). Although the extent of the child's disquiet and tension may be disproportionate to the problem, such a response may pose a risk for the child, thus indicating the need for therapy. On the other hand, a child who was involved in a traffic accident, traumatic experience, or difficult illness and whose parents believe is in deep need of therapy may be coping well emotionally despite mild symptoms, suggesting a contraindication to therapy. This question hones in on personal, individual differences among children.

Treatment Variables

The fourth and last consideration in this process of deciding on the need for therapy consists of treatment variables, including the prognosis and the relationship potential (Ronen, 1997b). Clinicians should ask themselves, from the existing knowledge available on the specific referred problem: Does it have a good prognosis? Is it worth investing efforts toward change? What is the likelihood of therapy rendering a change? Will the child be different after therapy? Can the child improve without therapy? And, from previous experience or the child's history: What are the chances of developing a good therapeutic relationship?

Here, it is important to assess and consider carefully previous therapeutic experiences. However, it is difficult to learn from them. A successful past treatment might hint at the child's ability to execute and comply with treatment assignments. However, unsuccessful past treatments may be attributable to other variables such as the child's younger age or the prior treatment techniques and plans, thus limiting the advisability of drawing conclusions about the child's relationship potential based on earlier nonsuccess.

The probability of spontaneous recovery for the specific referred problem needs to be weighed against the known success rates for its treatment. Often, even when the child does not express motivation but treatment is likely to resolve the problem, reaching out techniques can be used to attempt to activate the child toward change. However, when the prognosis for a problem is only fair and the child unmotivated, there is a need to look for other ways (e.g. environmental change) to help the child.

The therapeutic relationship is a major component for increasing motivation. Children usually attain better grades in classes where they like the teacher. Likewise, feelings of trust, confidence, and motivation in the therapeutic relationship will increase children's cooperation, help them invest more effort, and empower them to try new experiences.

The above four sets of variables are interconnected and must be evaluated integratively. For example, even if a problem is severe, its prognosis is not good, and the family does not support the change, but the child has motivation and can develop a good therapeutic relationship, an attempt at therapy may be worthwhile.

PHASE 2: HOW TO CLASSIFY CHILDREN'S REFERRALS AND GOALS FOR CHANGE

Assuming that the first phase of decision making led to the conclusion that a referred child's problem does warrant treatment, preliminary hypotheses have been formulated relating to the diagnosis. Now, the therapist enters the second phase of decision making. This phase centers on classifying referred problems according to their inherent goals for change and according to developmental stages, in order to facilitate the planning of assessment and treatment (Ronen, 2001).

The cognitive–behavioral orientation is a systematic approach that works toward clear, structured, attainable goals. Not only does its theoretical approach dictate working toward aims, but also the mutual client–therapist planning of targets, definition of expectations for change, and evaluation of achievements following intervention are major factors in the credo of the approach. The mutuality of the client–therapist decision making emphasizes the collaborative nature of the therapeutic contract, which directs the evolution of the treatment process (Rosenbaum & Ronen, 1998). By defining attainable goals, we empower clients, developing their belief in their own abilities and their sense of self-efficacy and confidence. This approach also educates and trains the client to adopt a problem-solving model for dealing with future problems. The client is thus taught to independently use the tools of defining realistic goals, examining expectations, working systematically toward achieving them, generating alternative means to reach these goals, and evaluating the extent of success. Defining targets and goals will elucidate what the treatment will focus on, which assessment tools should be selected, what setting is optimal, which techniques will best suit each target, and what evaluation and maintenance methods are preferred.

Therefore, when the therapist encounters a new referral, a decision should first be made regarding the long-term goals and expectations for the child, in terms of the four most common types of referral delineated below. Subsequently, intermediate goals can be defined to guide the therapeutic process, in terms of focusing on behavioral, emotional, cognitive, physiological, environmental, or interpersonal aspects. Finally, developmental stages must be considered in any classification of childhood referrals.

Long-Term Goal Classification

The literature highlights four prevalent types of referral in terms of their inherent treatment goals (Ronen, 1995, 1997b, 2001): (a) to decrease behaviors that the child exhibits too frequently, (b) to increase behaviors that the child does not exhibit often enough, (c) to remove anxieties that generate avoidance behavior, and (d) to facilitate developmental processes. Table 4.2 describes children's four most common types of referral in terms of their expected long-term goals in treatment, delineating the classification, behavioral examples, and the main immediate intervention targets involved in each type of treatment, as well as the assessment tools recommended for each referral type. Often children do not suffer from one sole problem, and there are many overlapping causes, kinds of problems, and types of treatment. This classification should therefore be used only for purposes of teaching, clarification, and emphasizing major trends.

The first types of referral are children who need to decrease behaviors. A lack of self-control skills and an impulsive style of thinking and acting distinguish these children. These "undercontrolled" children (Mash & Terdal, 1988) evidence difficulties in tolerating frustration, resisting temptation, delaying gratification, maintaining attention on target, or utilizing problem-solving skills. They often act

Table 4.2. Phase 2: Classification and Assessment of Children's Referrals and Goals for Change

Types of referral/goal			
Decrease behavior	Increase behavior	Remove anxiety	Facilitate development
Classification			
Undercontrolled Acting-out	Overcontrolled Acting-in	Overcontrolled Acting-in	Immature Childish
Behavior examples			
Impulsive Disobedient Aggressive	Depressed Shy Lonely	Fearful Phobic Overanxious	Crying Dependent
Characteristics			
Lack of self-control Impulsive thinking and acting	Low level of self-confidence and self-esteem	Avoidance of social situations	Inability to restrain or delay temptation
Immediate treatment targets			
Learn to tolerate frustration and delay temptation	Learn to set appropriate expectations & criteria Open up to new experiences	Acquire coping skills Open up to new experiences	Acquire mature skills
Assessment tools			
Parent and teacher reports Direct observation	Child's self-reports Standard emotional questionnaires	Child's self-monitoring Parent interview on child behavior	Developmental questionnaires Parent, teacher reports Direct observation

without thinking or planning, and, in situations where thinking would be beneficial, they lack careful information processing (Kendall, 1993).

In contrast, the second type of referral comprises children who need to increase their behaviors. Emotional dysfunction and a low level of self-confidence, self-acceptance, or self-esteem characterize them. These "overcontrolled" children (Mash & Terdal, 1988) often overemphasize self-evaluation, frequently establishing overly high goals or criteria for themselves and thereby underappreciating their own achievements. Kendall (1993) described such children as limited to distorted thinking, where they misconstrue and misconceive social situations. Thus, interventions with these children should address distortions in their self-concept and should challenge them to do more, with a focus on experiencing and practicing.

When children suffer from anxiety (the third type of referral), they cannot achieve their potential capacities due to the avoidance and regression produced by their fears, anxieties, and trauma. These overcontrolled children should accumulate a wider repertoire of coping skills and should practice exposure assignments that would enable them to try out new experiences.

Children whose development needs to be facilitated due to their immaturity comprise the last type of referral. They need help in stopping childish behaviors such as the tendency to cry too often, learning to restrain themselves, taking on responsibility for their behavior, and trying to delay satisfaction or overcome temptation. Treatment for these children should promote the acquisition of new, mature skills, furnish practice in new tasks, and supply new models for change. The environment is of great importance for facilitating a child's development, for example, in families where the child's immature behavior may stem not only from a lack of skills, but also from a lack of opportunity in the family for the child to be independent or take on responsibilities.

It should be emphasized that while considering the expected intermediate targets of intervention (e.g. behaviors, emotions, and/or cognitions), one should remember that no change is exclusively behavioral, emotional, cognitive, or interpersonal in its nature (Shirk & Russell, 1996). Interrelations exist between all realms, with mutual effects; therefore, intervening in one realm precipitates changes in the others. For example, a boy in behavior therapy who is working on improving his low academic achievement (cognitive focus) will also gain an emotional change by increasing his self-confidence and self-esteem. A girl with encopresis who is working through art therapy on letting go and withholding, to change her emotions and self-acceptance, will also improve her behavior and change her toileting habits. Or, a boy referred to therapy due to his lack of assertiveness may receive a behavioral treatment including training in standing still, talking loudly, and maintaining direct eye contact (Bandura, 1969, 1997), but not only will behavioral changes transpire but also emotional fluctuations. His enactment of a self-confident posture will generate an increased feeling of security and confidence.

The Impact of Problem Type on the Selection of Assessment Tools

As seen in Table 4.2, the choice of assessment tools is influenced by the classification into these four referral types as well. Careful decision making on the types of assessment measures should be based on the child's problem, the child's referral, and the goals of therapy. The predominant methods for child assessment are based on psychological tests (verbal, association) and projective testing (drawing, reflecting), which inquire into the child's internal world (Goldman et al., 1983). Although there is no right or wrong measurement among the variety of assessment tools available, a standard, familiar battery of tests is usually administered, without much consideration of individual needs. Clinicians should become more accustomed to asking themselves: What impact does the type of problem presented by the child have on selecting particular assessment tools?

In selecting appropriate modes of assessment, the main objective for the therapist to keep in mind is that tools should be elected to obtain different information. For example, when the child evidences undercontrolled behavior, we need to learn about the severity of specific disorders (e.g. conduct disorder). In such cases, administering a specific inventory or scale (e.g. Achenbach & Edelbrock, 1983; Conners, 1969; Eyberg, 1980) to the parents or teacher would be in order. However, when a child exhibits overcontrolled behavior, such as loneliness and a poor social behavior pattern, direct observation of the child's behavior in the natural setting, or daily records maintained by the child, might be the assessment method of choice. When the child suffers from an anxiety disorder (the third type of referral) and we wish to learn about the child's emotional state, it is better to directly test the child or ask the child to report about internal states. In this case, projective methods are the method of choice. When the child exhibits immature behavior, a developmental test might be helpful for comparing the child's behavior to environmental criteria.

Another consideration would be which source of information is the most reliable for that specific type of disorder (see Chapter 1). While parents are the most reliable source for learning about acting-out disorders, they are not reliable to report about children's internal behavior. Children's self-reports would be more appropriate for learning about acting-in disorders. The other chief objective for clinicians is to select assessment tools in order to facilitate the intervention's goals. The clinician should ask: How will this specific assessment tool change the way I plan to intervene with the child? Will its different outcomes point to the need for different kinds of intervention settings, treatment methods, or techniques to be used?

Intermediate Goal Classification

All problems have behavioral, cognitive, and emotional aspects. When we define intermediate targets (as illustrated in Table 4.2), we are selecting specific aspects for intervention at a particular stage of treatment. For example, in treating a boy who exhibits violent behavior, we will typically define his problem as a behavior that needs to be decreased, and we will usually work mainly using behavioral methods, primarily through the environment (via parent and/or teacher counseling). However, the violent child suffers from emotional problems related to frustration, emotional regulation, and aggression, requiring individual work. At the same time, such a child's interpersonal problems will probably necessitate group work to improve social skills. And, sometimes, cognitive work must precede any of these interventions, in order to change the boy's basic thinking patterns comprising hostile and negative perceptions of the world in which he lives. Therefore, when classifying behavior in this context, our aim is not the child's diagnosis, but rather defining the specific aspects or parts of the child's behavior that need attention and intervention.

Referred Problem Classification According to Developmental Considerations

In weighing children's referrals and establishing treatment goals, the classification proposed above employing four problem types with their long-term and intermediate goals can provide a solid framework, but it is incomplete without taking into account the developmental components that are part and parcel of child intervention. Table 4.3 presents a second type of classification paradigm, based on the characteristics of children's referral, assessment, treatment, evaluation, and maintenance in terms of four major developmental stages: infancy, early childhood, middle childhood, and adolescence. This classification aims to complement the problem classification by focusing on developmental issues. As can be seen in Table 4.3, children's referrals can be classified into different kinds of problems that depend on the cognitive level (Piaget, 1924) as well as the expected social tasks (Forehand & Weirson, 1993) characterizing the four developmental stages. Again, this classification should serve only as a general paradigm to clarify major trends for educational purposes.

Forehand and Weirson (1993) linked treatment planning with the new roles and social tasks evident at each developmental age or stage. Infants' major developmental task involves a shift from total dependence on the caregiver to increased independence and self-regulation, producing a range of normal educational and developmental difficulties. In toddlerhood and then early childhood (ages 3–5), the major developmental task, beginning mastery of academic and social situations, generates behavioral and discipline problems. Middle childhood (ages 6–11) is focused on the task of cultivating personal identity and self-control, thereby leading to problems in self-control and interpersonal difficulties. Finally, in adolescence (12–18), the major developmental tasks comprise separation and individuation from the family. This phase precipitates problems in establishing

Table 4.3. Phase 2: Children's Problems and Their Assessment Based on Developmental Stages

	Stages			
	Infancy (0–2 years)	Early childhood (3–5 years)	Middle childhood (6–11 years)	Adolescence (12–18 years)
Cognitive level	Motoric and basic cognitive skills	Concrete pre-operational thinking	Concrete operational thinking	Abstract thinking
Social tasks	Shift from dependence to increased independence	Mastery of academic and social situations	Cultivating personal identity & self-control	Separation & individuation from the family
Main problems	Normal educational & developmental difficulties	Behavioral & discipline problems Interpersonal difficulties	Problems in self-control	Problems in identity, autonomy regulation, and family interaction
Assessment tools	Parent reports on behavior	Parent & teacher reports	Child testing Peer reports	Family reports Self-reports Teacher reports

a personal identity, regulating one's sense of autonomy, and interacting within the family.

As seen in Table 4.3, the selection of assessment methods should also be made on the basis of the child's age and developmental stage. Emphasis should be placed on the child's cognitive level, expected social tasks, and the value of different information sources at various developmental stages. Clinicians should thus become accustomed to asking themselves: Which kind of assessment will best address the presented questions being posed about this specific child at this specific age?

PHASE 3: HOW TO DECIDE WHO SHOULD BE TREATED (SETTING) BASED ON DEVELOPMENTAL VARIABLES AND REFERRAL TYPE

The next issue for therapists to contemplate, following the classification of children's referrals and goals of change, concerns how the child's developmental stage and referral type should influence the treatment setting. Or, in other words, how should one decide who should be the targeted client system to be treated?

When an adult is referred to therapy, as a general rule we conduct individual therapy with that client, and occasionally we may recommend marital or family intervention. However, when a child is referred, many alternative therapeutic settings are available from which to choose. We can supervise the child's parents or teachers in a group setting aimed at skill acquisition, or we may counsel them individually toward the specific change needed with that particular child (Ronen, 1992, 1993b,c, 2001). We can implement family therapy, involving all members of the family (or only some, as in dyadic therapy) and focusing on roles, relationships, and communication patterns. Or, we may choose to treat the child's classroom or treat the child in group therapy. And, finally, we have the option of applying individual therapy with the child (Kazdin, 1988a).

In order to decide on the optimal intervention setting, decisions should be based on several main features: the child's developmental characteristics, the kind of problem referred, and the child's individual characteristics.

Developmental Variables

As briefly outlined in Chapter 1, the child's developmental features have a major impact on the intervention setting selection. At different ages, children have different social roles and different capabilities (Forehand & Weirson, 1993). As can be seen in Table 4.4, developmental variables thus influence the decision regarding who should be treated.

Table 4.4. Phase 3: Selecting Appropriate Setting(s) Based on Developmental Stage

	Stages			
	Infancy (0–2 years)	Early childhood (3–5 years)	Middle childhood (6–11 years)	Adolescence (12–18 years)
Intervention setting	Counseling environment (parents)	Counseling environment (with child)	Child in individual, group, or family	Individual therapy Peer group Family therapy

During infancy and early toddlerhood, when children are young and dependent on their caregivers, difficulties in achieving initial gains in autonomy usually derive from parents' educational practices. Therefore, therapy up to the age of 2 years usually has primary prevention aims (i.e. preventing future risk and reducing the incidence of disorder, Graham, 1994) and takes the form of counseling and supervising parents in educating and rearing their children (Ronen, 1997b, 2001). As children grow into early childhood, they encounter the academic and social tasks inherent in preschool experience. Interventions at this time most often involve parent and teacher supervision (preferably in the children's presence) concerning their relationships and discipline methods. Children of this age are seldom treated directly. Thus, from the ages of 3 to 5, therapy should be directed to the child within his or her natural environment (i.e. parents, teachers, and friends). Also, it is directed toward educational–therapeutic tasks in keeping with secondary prevention goals (i.e. which prevent existing problems from worsening and reduce the duration of the disorder, Graham, 1994).

From the ages of 6 through 11, in middle childhood and preadolescence, the child searches for personal identity and the acquisition of self-control. These tasks suggest the need to implement individual or group therapy focusing on social support, self-evaluation, and acceptance.

As children enter middle adolescence, the developmental tasks at hand comprise individuation from the family unit and a move toward autonomy. These tasks require direct intervention with the adolescent to promote individualization, self-acceptance, and problem solving skills. Thus, from the age of 12, youngsters' therapy should focus on tertiary prevention, which aims to resolve an already existing problem, prevent future risks or disability arising from an established disorder, impart skills for decreasing its frequency, and cover rehabilitative activities (Graham, 1994). As can be seen, children should generally be treated not with a focus on one setting only, but rather on a combination of settings that considers developmental factors. Thus, age and cognitive stage can be seen to dictate the kind of intervention setting best suited to a child; however, the therapist's determination must also take into account characteristics of the specific problem inducing referral.

Problem Variables

The selection of the optimal setting for intervention is also influenced by the type of children's referrals with their long-term and intermediate goals (Ronen, 2001). An example of how a problem may influence the setting would be a social skills deficit. Such a deficit necessitates acquiring specific skills that can best be fostered in groups, where the child can experience and practice the desired behavior. If the intermediate target is interpersonal, the most efficient setting may be interpersonal in nature (e.g. group therapy, family therapy). If the intermediate target is emotional, the setting will be individual, and the intervention technique will be more expressive and experimental. Table 4.5 depicts how the four common referral types in terms of their long-term goals can offer general guidelines for determining the optimal setting.

Generally, children who exhibit acting-out disorders (needing to decrease behaviors) usually do not suffer from their problems to the extent that the environment suffers. Thus, individual therapy with such children is usually not as effective as treatments directed toward a change in the environment's response to the child, as well as toward changing the environment itself. Therefore, for undercontrolled children, the main target of intervention is usually the supervision of parents or teachers or the application of family therapy.

On the other hand, when a child has overcontrolled behaviors that need to be increased in frequency, emotional features are often prominent. Therapy can facilitate the child's expression of emotions; ability to overcome fears, depression, and guilt; amelioration of negative self-evaluations; and development of a sense of self-efficacy and self-confidence (Ronen, 1998b). The target of intervention for acting-in children, therefore, is mainly individual or group therapy for the child. Secondarily, supervising or counseling the environment may be needed.

In treating the third kind of problem, difficulties related to anxiety and fears, the child must be helped to express emotions, to practice exposure to the feared situations, and to be supported by the environment. The main settings for

Table 4.5. Phase 3: Selecting the Targeted Client Setting Based on Type of Referral

	Types of referral			
	Decrease behavior (Undercontrolled)	Increase behavior (Overcontrolled)	Remove anxiety (Overcontrolled)	Facilitate development (Immature)
Intervention setting	Parent counseling	Individual therapy	Child therapy (with parents)	Parent and kindergarten teacher counseling
	Parent therapy (with child)	Group therapy		

children referred with this type of problem are individual child therapy to impart the needed skills for change, along with parent counseling to enhance environmental support.

When the expected goal of therapy at referral is to facilitate development, the child's environment must come into the forefront of intervention. Although sometimes there is a need to directly impart the immature child with mature skills, such skills are typically acquired via environmental change. Parents can learn to increase demands, to give the child added tasks, roles, and responsibilities in the family, and to reinforce positive behavior as well. The kindergarten or elementary school teacher can learn how to reinforce a mature behavior and ignore a childish one. Peers can play a role by becoming involved in helping the child learn new roles and behaviors.

It can be seen, then, that as a general rule, when a child is young in age or demonstrates behavior problems (which require decreasing behaviors or facilitating development), the environment is typically targeted for intervention (e.g. parent counseling). On the other hand, when a child is in middle childhood and up or suffers from emotional problems (which require increasing behaviors or removing anxiety), the targeted client system is usually the child himself or herself (i.e. individual intervention, usually along with parent counseling).

Child Variables

The unique nature of each child is the last variable that must be taken into consideration when making a decision as to which client(s) should be targeted for treatment. For example, let us look at a case of a 6-year-old boy. At this age, he has just emerged from the pre-operational stage. Treatment at this age is usually nonverbal and indirect and involves parents; however, if the child is very intelligent, has advanced verbal skills, and is highly motivated to learn, cognitive–constructivist individual verbal therapy can be applied.

PHASE 4: CREATIVE THINKING IN SELECTING APPROPRIATE MODES AND TECHNIQUES FOR CHANGE

Up to now, we have decided whether or not the presented problem necessitates therapy, how the child's referral and therapeutic goals can be classified and assessed, and later on, who should be treated and in what setting, all the while incorporating developmental considerations. The next question, therefore, is how therapy should be applied.

Children have traditionally been treated using nonverbal, indirect therapeutic modes such as play therapy (Axline, 1947). However, the increased application of cognitive therapies with children has opened up the direct and verbal modes to child therapists (Knell, 1993). The recent constructivist branch of cognitive therapy (Mahoney, 1991; Neimeyer & Mahoney, 1995) highlights the importance of integrating various techniques into the process of change, and this approach has become more popular over the last decade. At the same time, the distinct parallels between treatment mode and theoretical orientation have blurred. For example, play therapy is no longer considered to be solely in the dominion of dynamic intervention, but rather can be applied in behavior therapy or cognitive therapy as well (Knell, 1993). Child therapists of diverse theoretical backgrounds (e.g. client-centered, dynamic, cognitive, behavioral, constructivist) now utilize a range of treatment techniques (whether play, drawing, discussion, imagery, etc.) by creatively adapting them to the clinicians' theoretical orientations (Ronen, 1994).

Therefore, when making decisions concerning the best way to design a child's treatment, the therapist's theoretical background is no longer the sole influence. To be sure, therapist preferences and characteristics are one of the four basic variables to be considered when selecting specific modes and techniques for intervention, along with child characteristics such as style and interests, developmental issues, and the nature of the referred problem (Knell, 1993; Ronen, 1992, 1993b). Yet, the role of the therapist here is to take all of these variables into account in order to creatively and flexibly introduce the optimal therapeutic modes and techniques.

Therapist Characteristics

The selection of methods for intervention crucially depends on the therapist's theoretical approach on the one hand, but also depends on the fact that each therapist has his or her own style. As an illustration, individuals who favor music can use their talents or knowledge in this domain to apply music therapy; other artistically inclined therapists would naturally seek out art or dance therapy (Mahoney, 1991). I even have a student, a clinical social worker, who studied the Shiatzu massage method and conducts a wonderful treatment program combining the Shiatzu method with cognitive therapy in working with prisoners. Another student of mine combines his knowledge of massage therapy with cognitive therapy to help people open up to experiences, in a method similar to that suggested by Mahoney (1991).

On the other hand, it is very difficult for therapists to conduct therapy using a technique with which they feel uncomfortable. For example, in teaching my graduate classes of social workers who specialize in child therapy, I always bring in an art therapist to do some hands-on creative work with my students. I believe that therapists should first try each creative technique on themselves before applying it to their clients (Ronen & Rosenbaum, 1998). On one occasion, a student who had previously demonstrated a readiness for self-examination and the ability to receive constructive criticism adamantly resisted the art therapist's assignment that she sculpt her own family. This student was simply not able to bring herself to participate in that class activity, claiming that it "wasn't her style." We may all prefer one technique over another, but I doubt if someone can be a truly good therapist if he or she resists practicing every new technique and always adheres to the old, routine methods in which he or she was trained. I believe it will be difficult for this aforementioned student to use sculpturing in her therapeutic work, and that is fine, if she will be ready to try other nonverbal methods and is aware of the reasons behind her avoidance.

Child Characteristics

It is very difficult to ask a child who hates to draw to take part in art therapy that has a drawing focus, and by selecting such a technique the therapist is likely to face rejection. On the other hand, for a boy who loves movies, his hobby can be used to ask him to write a new scene depicting how his behavior will look in the future. Similarly, a girl who writes poetry can create a poem about her life. For example, I treated a girl who had previously been hospitalized for several years because of anorexia (Ronen & Ayelet, 2001). Her hospital therapists had claimed that her lack of cooperation in arts and crafts sessions was an impediment to her recovery. However, this girl was very talented artistically. She did indeed refuse to participate in the hospital's art sessions because she found them extremely dull. Yet, she showed me a profuse portfolio from that period of time, when she had been writing moving poetry and creating wonderfully expressive drawings. If someone had listened to her carefully, that abundance of creative work could have been used as an effective tool to learn more about this girl and to help her change.

Several years ago, I interviewed a mother and her 14-year-old obese son. The mother was concerned about his health and wanted me to treat him for his eating disorder, but he resisted therapy. He and I made a contract that he would come to one individual session and then we would decide how to proceed. During that session, I discovered that he was very interested in playing basketball and felt badly about failing to participate in this game. We made an agreement to start self-control therapy for improving his basketball skills. We spent most of the sessions outside, playing basketball and identifying the methods most useful to him. Only much later was he ready to start talking about his weight and to transfer the learned self-control skills to the area of his eating disorder.

Developmental Issues

The age, sex, and major developmental (cognitive and social) tasks facing the child must be of prime concern in designing treatment. As described in Chapter 1, specific developmental processes and opportunities may emerge differentially for boys and girls and for children at different ages and stages of development, suggesting that diverse interventions are necessary to achieve change accordingly

Table 4.6. Phase 4: Selecting Treatment Methods Based on Developmental Stages

	Stages			
	Infancy (0–2 years)	Early childhood (3–5 years)	Middle childhood (6–11 years)	Adolescence (12–18 years)
Main treatment methods	Verbal therapy (adults)	Verbal therapy (parents or family) Nonverbal (child)	Indirect and/or direct therapy (child)	Direct verbal therapy

(Kazdin, 1994b). Even while conducting cognitive–constructivist therapy, it is possible to select various treatment techniques that should discriminate between developmental factors and be adaptable to children based on their abilities. Table 4.6 presents general guidelines for choosing treatment methods based on the child's developmental stage.

In general, infants and young children are not usually treated directly, but rather their parents are supervised through verbal communication in how to change their children's behavior. Young children (before the age of 6), who are at the concrete stage of thinking and have limited verbal ability, can benefit more from indirect treatment and mostly from nonverbal techniques such as playing or drawing. Between the ages of 6 and 11, in the school years, when children become candidates for group or individual treatment, they may certainly start to benefit from verbal therapy. However, due to schoolchildren's continued use of concrete thinking and their limited perceptions of time, morality, and world concepts, verbal treatments at this age should include many indirect methods such as examples, demonstrations, writing, reading, and bibliotherapy. Nonverbal techniques can also still be effective, such as music, movement, and sculpture. Only in adolescence does most therapy become verbal and direct, involving teenagers in talking about the issues of most concern to them. At this stage, youngsters can participate in a wider range of treatments, including verbal, nonverbal, direct, and indirect methods. Cognitive–constructivist therapy can best be applied combining such indirect verbal techniques as imagery and metaphor with direct discussion (Kopp, 1995).

Problem Variables

The selection of the appropriate therapeutic methods and techniques for children will take into account a number of referral and assessment variables. These include the characteristics of the child's specific disorder, the kinds of behaviors and deficits presented, and the negative impact these have caused to the child and/or to his or her environment. As can be seen in Table 4.7, the optimal

Table 4.7. Phase 4: Therapeutic Methods Based on the Four Types of Referral

Goal of therapy	Decreasing behavior (Under-controlled)	Increasing behavior (Over-controlled)	Removing anxiety (Over-controlled)	Facilitating development (Immature)
Kind of therapy	Verbal supervision	Nonverbal & verbal	Experiential & verbal	Verbal & practicing

treatment method should be selected only after the careful identification of the referred problem type and thus the treatment's expected goal (i.e. decreasing a behavior, increasing a behavior, removing anxiety, or facilitating development).

Internal, emotional difficulties (e.g. depression, anxiety, and self-esteem) have been defined by Achenbach (1985), Mash and Terdal (1988), and Kendall and Braswell (1985) as overcontrolled problems. Those emotional disorders are characterized by distorted thinking. The treatment of choice for emotional disorders is emotion-focused experiential therapy using a nonverbal and indirect treatment mode. On the other hand, while treating externalizing or undercontrolled problems (e.g. aggression, disobedience, and hyperactivity), a more direct, verbal therapeutic mode is recommended.

PHASE 5: HOW TO EVALUATE AND MAINTAIN TREATMENT OUTCOMES

The ultimate goal of child psychotherapy is to gain a curative effect, whether in the form of achieving behavioral improvement, emotional change, or symptomatic relief, or in the form of learning needed skills or increasing independent functioning in the future. Accordingly, the evaluation of the treatment's outcome must be an integral part of any intervention. Evaluation methods significantly assist therapists in learning about an individual's state after treatment, a particular change process, or the efficacy of a specific intervention (Kazdin, 1982, 1994a). Research on treatment outcomes may consider general group changes or single case designs that examine individual differences and process issues.

The therapist's selection of evaluation methods should be based on the treatment goal as well as on developmental considerations. Customarily, evaluation should appraise changes that occurred both in the child and in the environment and should compare reports from different sources to obtain a comprehensive picture (Achenbach, 1993). As presented in Table 4.8, the evaluation of treatment outcomes should take into account the goal of therapy, in terms of the four most common types of child referrals.

Table 4.8. Phase 5: Evaluating Treatment Outcomes Based on the Four Types of Referral

Goal of therapy	Decreasing behavior (Under-controlled)	Increasing behavior (Over-controlled)	Removing anxiety (Over-controlled)	Facilitating development (Immature)
Evaluation methods	Behavior change Reports from environment on functioning	Child reports on social relations and emotions	Child and parent reports on behavior	Parent and teacher reports Observation

I do not relate to evaluation measurement as a separate entity, because the best way to evaluate children's progress is to compare their behavior at the end of therapy with that at the beginning of or prior to therapy. It is therefore important to use the same assessment tools in outcome evaluation as in initial baseline assessment. If baseline assessment and diagnosis comprised parents' reports or teacher reports, it is valuable to return to these information sources and ask again for their input. If the child's behavior was initially observed directly, the best way to evaluate progress would be to repeat the observation procedure. In cases where children completed empirical tests at the baseline stage, those tests can be re-administered. Often, a good evaluation method constitutes the use of ongoing self-reports and records that the child and the parents maintain throughout the process of therapy. I often ask children to assess and evaluate their own situation themselves. I also use these records to tangibly demonstrate to children those changes that they have succeeded in accomplishing. When children are capable of analyzing the difference between baseline functioning and end-of-therapy functioning, it is highly likely that these self-reports can serve an empowering function that encourages children to continue investing effort into achieving improvement.

Three main areas must be emphasized by treatment evaluation. First, behavior change is assessed to determine if the disorder that prompted the child's referral has been eliminated. Behavioral questionnaires using self-report and parent or teacher reports can provide this information. Second, emotional change should be evaluated, approaching the child as the primary source of information. Research has demonstrated that parents are good sources for evaluating children's behavior but not their emotions (Angold et al., 1987; Hodges et al., 1990; Reid et al., 1987). Emotional information can be gleaned from verbal self-report questionnaires (e.g. on anxiety, loneliness, depression, etc.) or through indirect, projective methods such as drawing or formal projective testing. Third, cognitive changes must be addressed. Perceptions, attitudes, and thinking styles can be directly measured through attitude scales, self-efficacy questionnaires, etc.

Maintenance of Treatment Outcomes

Cognitive–behavioral therapy does not end at termination, at the time that significant progress has been evaluated by a comparison to baseline functioning. Rather, therapy includes a crucial follow-up stage with the express goal of teaching skills to maintain the treatment outcomes that have been achieved. In other words, cognitive–behavioral therapy not only strongly emphasizes the initial process of changing the problem, but also accentuates the enormous importance of relapse prevention and maintenance of changes after the specific problem has been resolved. It is during the follow-up period that work must continue to enable the client's newly learned, desired, mediated behaviors to gradually become automatic and habitual. Clients must be taught to continue self-monitoring in order to identify signs of impending regression and must be prepared for the inevitability of the ups and downs characterizing human emotion and behavior. Self-reinforcement and a sense of autonomy must be fostered to assist the client in coping with future challenges and setbacks.

In order to achieve maintenance, therapy must routinely utilize specific techniques and components to preserve the treatment outcomes. These components include prevention of regression, overlearning, generalization, and transfer of learned skills in order to develop future independent functioning (Kanfer & Schefft, 1988; Ronen, 1997b). Follow-up procedures for self-evaluation, such as the continued, systematic self-monitoring, recording, and charting of targeted behaviors even after regular treatment sessions are discontinued, can facilitate a sense of commitment, control, and responsibility and, simultaneously, serve as a reminder to continue applying learned skills and tools. During this stage, skills and exercises that have already been mastered (e.g. generating mediated, positive thoughts instead of automatic, negative ones) should nevertheless continue to be practiced until the point of overlearning, when the learned behavior becomes habitual and automatic. To enhance the transfer and generalization necessary to develop independence in the future, Ronen and Rosenbaum (2001) have developed a systematic self-control intervention model that invites a child who has resolved one problem under the therapist's full guidance to then select another problem for self-help.

The duration of the follow-up period and the frequency and type of contact recommended between therapists and clients during that period are a direct function of treatment duration, problem severity, and developmental variables. In terms of treatment duration, as a general rule, long-term interventions necessitate a longer follow-up period than do short-term interventions. Likewise, a more severe problem generally necessitates a longer maintenance period to ensure that the client has genuinely overcome the disorder and is capable of coping better independently. Mild problems and, usually, short-term interventions are easier to terminate after one or two follow-up sessions. Long-term interventions and more severe disorders may require a follow-up period lasting up to several months.

As can be seen in Table 4.9, with regard to developmental variables, a younger child needs frequent, brief follow-up sessions such as weekly telephone sessions, or weekly 10-minute follow-up meetings in person. Older children can function more independently while maintaining contact with the therapist once every 2–3 weeks, or, for adolescents, every 3–4 weeks. In either case, the frequency of the follow-up sessions ideally decreases gradually, although, as I will mention below, in many cases contact is terminated abruptly by the client.

The selection of optimal follow-up techniques should consider both developmental components and the targeted aspects of the problem necessitating continued maintenance. Various techniques can be used at different ages to maintain treatment outcomes, as seen in Table 4.9. For example, in the treatment of infants, where therapy is usually conducted via parental supervision, useful follow-up techniques include parents' self-recording and charting of behaviors. Gradually, parents are advised to desist from this process of keeping written records. In early childhood, treatment is usually directed toward parents and children. Here, short follow-up sessions or frequent telephone calls are important to reinforce the family and to facilitate the generalization and transfer of achievements to other problem areas. In middle childhood, when children are treated directly, techniques of overlearning are crucial to strengthen skills and prevent

Table 4.9. Follow Up and Maintenance of Treatment Outcomes

Developmental stage	Client setting	Follow-up frequency	Follow-up techniques
Infancy	Parent supervision	Every 3–4 weeks	Self-recording Charting Self-reinforcement
Early childhood	Child and family	Weekly telephone calls or brief sessions	Charting Reinforcements Gradual withdrawal from treatment conditions
Middle childhood	Child	Every 2–3 weeks	Role playing Generalization Skills transfer Overlearning
Adolescence	Child	Every 3–4 weeks	Skills practice Overlearning Role-playing Relapse prevention Generalization

regression. Role-playing can also help children rehearse their newly acquired skills to prepare them for applying the skills in other problem areas and situations. Similarly, adolescents can learn to prevent relapse through role-playing by practicing how they might behave in difficult situations in the future. For instance: "Let's imagine that you're arguing with your parents. How would you control yourself then?" or "What will you do next time you feel you're too tired to get up and go to school?" or "What will you think to yourself next time a friend doesn't smile at you when you think he should?" Overlearning, generalization, and skills practice complement such activities.

The selection of optimal maintenance techniques also depends on the identification of those aspects of the client's problems that are being targeted in the follow-up period. Usually, when a client improves dramatically during treatment, many changes occur in all areas of their lives, in terms of how the environment regards them, how they relate to their surroundings, and how they view themselves and feel about themselves. Thus, these changes and improvements essentially reinforce continued success, both internally and interpersonally. In these cases when the changes have implications on the environment, regardless of whether the difficulties stem from an undercontrolled behavior such as violence or from overcontrolled behaviors such as depressive withdrawal or social problems, the changes evident in the client due to therapy automatically lead to changes in interpersonal relations. For example, the teacher will naturally reinforce the improved child for better behavior, and other children will want to spend more time with the child, inviting him or her to be in their company more often. Therefore, such problems usually do not require controlled techniques during follow up, because the environment has undergone training and is already naturally reinforcing desired behavior and facilitating the maintenance of improvement. Follow up can be shorter, and can focus on the client report about the achievements that are maintained.

On the other hand, in cases where the problems lie within the person, relating to issues of self-esteem or private issues (e.g. enuresis), follow-up sessions should emphasize explicit, controlled relapse prevention techniques, self-recording, and overlearning in order to make sure the client now has the proper skills to cope with obstacles and difficulties.

Follow-up sessions should be conducted as long as clients feel uncertain about their ability to preserve their achievements and to cope independently with what lies ahead, or until the therapist is confident that the client is continuing to employ skills appropriately, coping autonomously, and maintaining treatment outcomes. However, the duration of the follow-up period significantly depends on the client's cooperation with this process. We must be realistic; once they have improved significantly, people are no longer highly motivated to continue therapy. Indeed, if the therapist is confident that a relapse will not ensue, he or she has a vested interest in gradually weaning clients from dependence on therapy, thus empowering clients, instilling dignity, self-respect, and pride in their success and autonomy.

I would like to add that, frequently, as the goals of therapy are achieved, children, and especially adolescents, are overwhelmingly relieved to be rid of their problems and oftentimes, now that they are functioning smoothly, feel intense shame that they could not control the problem on their own before. In their eagerness to detach themselves from the therapy that reminds them of their previous distress, they may prefer not to comply with follow-up sessions and to end the maintenance stage prematurely (in the therapist's eyes). We cannot coerce clients to attend follow-up sessions, but we must remember that during treatment we have given them the tools to maintain progress and to identify signs of regression. Moreover, the beneficial effect of ending therapy on self-esteem is often tremendous. What I do try to do is to reinforce the client for his or her confidence and progress, thus empowering the client to believe in his or her own capabilities. At the same time, I offer an open door policy, asking them not to wait or hesitate if they wish to call me for consultation or to share anything with me.

* * *

In sum, as can be seen in this chapter, cognitive–constructivist therapy entails a constant process of decision making about what should be the treatment of choice (including assessment, diagnosis, treatment, evaluation, and maintenance) for that specific client, with that specific problem, at this specific stage of life, and with his or her own personal characteristics.

5

Self-Control Therapy with Children

Chapter 4 described assessment, treatment, evaluation, and maintenance considerations for applying cognitive–constructivist therapy with children. In the scenario where, via these guidelines, it was decided that therapy was necessary and that the child could benefit from individual therapy, in general, and from cognitive–constructivist therapy, in particular, this chapter describes the content of my self-control intervention model that can be applied to children.

Child therapy is a combination of art and skill. Skill is needed to select the appropriate cognitive–constructivist techniques in designing the intervention process, whereas the artistic ability refers to the therapist's creative adaptation of his or her basic theory to the child's age, stage, problems, personality, and environment. In this chapter, I will try to elucidate how child treatment can be conducted.

One of the most popular cognitive–constructivist treatments for children is self-control training. The present chapter reviews some of the existing self-control therapies and then proposes a self-control intervention model for treating childhood disorders.

IMPARTING CHILDREN WITH SELF-CONTROL SKILLS

Self-control has become a popular intervention method with children because it comprises a main target in therapy as well as in education. Enabling a child to control himself or herself is one of the primary goals of teachers, educators, counselors, and parents. On the other side of the coin, many childhood disorders relate to the area of self-control, whether the child suffers from a lack of self-control or cannot relinquish control.

The basic ideas underlying self-control interventions are that human behavior is goal directed, always in a process of changing and developing, and associated with interactive factors that influence the process of self-regulating behavior (Kanfer & Schefft, 1988; Karoly & Kanfer, 1982; Rosenbaum, 1990, 1993). Learning is considered to play a central role in the acquisition and maintenance of a behavior, whether adaptive or dysfunctional (Kendall, 1993, 1994; Mash & Terdal, 1988). Self-control skills are not in use in everyday behavior. These are skills needed when one faces difficulties, when obstacles need to be overcome to achieve goals, when new behaviors need to be learned, when choices need to be made, or when habitual response sequences are interrupted or prove ineffective (Kanfer & Schefft, 1988).

Self-control training is based on the client's active participation, in learning to look at irrational thoughts, stopping automatic thoughts, changing them to mediated ones, starting an internal dialogue, and looking for alternative behaviors (Beck et al., 1979; Copeland, 1982; Meichenbaum, 1979, 1985; Ronen, 1994, 1997a,b). With children, self-control training does not constitute a comprehensive intervention method, but instead comprises an umbrella term for a large variety of treatment techniques. Through these self-control techniques, children are taught to use cognitive mediational strategies to guide their behavior and thus improve their adjustment (Durlak et al., 1991; Kendall, 1993). The main goal of change is skills acquisition (Karoly & Kanfer, 1982; Ronen, 1997a,b; Rosenbaum, 1990), focusing on the immediate goal of solving children's behavior problems. The targets of self-control interventions have included interpersonal thinking, means–end thinking, planning and anticipating skills, self-instruction, coping with stress, inhibiting responses, self-reinforcement, and use of problem-solving methods (Cowen, 1980; Elias et al., 1986; Kendall, 1993; Ronen, 1997b). The range of different disorders that have been treated by self-control training includes: impulsivity and hyperactivity (Kendall & Braswell, 1985; Kendall & Wilcox, 1980; Meichenbaum & Goodman, 1971); aggression (Kazdin, 1987; Kazdin et al., 1987); disobedience and disruptiveness problems (Copeland, 1982; Gross & Drabman, 1982); depression (Kazdin, 1988b, 1994b); and fears and anxieties (Kanfer et al., 1975; Kendall, 1994; Ronen, 1996b).

These programs all aimed at teaching children how to use self-instruction, cope with stress, inhibit disadvantageous responses, reinforce themselves, and use problem-solving methods; and they included training in techniques such as self-talk, self-evaluation, self-monitoring, and thinking aloud (Elias et al., 1986; Kendall & Braswell, 1985). The acquisition of self-control skills promotes the child's ability to identify his or her automatic, habitual way of thinking and change it into a mediated, planned way of thinking. Self-control skills facilitate children's recognition of the role of thought in emotional arousal, empowering them to overcome disturbing emotions, to learn the causes of their behavior, and to acquire effective techniques for behavioral change (Copeland, 1982; Kendall & Braswell, 1985; Meichenbaum, 1979; Ronen et al., 1992, 1995; Ronen & Wozner, 1995).

Controlled studies have been conducted on self-control interventions in the area of fears and anxieties (Barrios & Hartman, 1988); hyperactivity and impulsivity (Kendall & Braswell, 1985); and disobedience and disruptiveness problems (Copeland, 1982; Gross & Drabman, 1982; Brigham et al., 1979). Those studies proved self-control training to be effective.

THE EFFICACY OF THE SELF-CONTROL INTERVENTION MODEL (SCIM) WITH CHILDREN

In line with the aforementioned theoretical and empirical literature, I have developed an intervention model aimed at teaching children self-control skills for solving their problems, whether externalizing or internalizing disorders. The model proposes an educational therapeutic process (Ronen & Wozner, 1995). Each phase increases progress toward the achievement of control over the behavior.

In trying to learn the influence of self-control skills on children's behavior, this treatment approach was found to be effective in achieving change for a wide range of problem areas. In some children, increasing general self-control skills affected problematic behaviors (e.g. a general training program in self-control for 12-year-old children led to an improvement in social skills, see Ronen, 1994). In other cases, it was necessary to impart children with specific, problem-related self-control skills in order to have a significant effect on decreasing problems (cf., Ronen et al., 1995).

The intervention model for changing children's behavior was originally applied to the treatment of enuretic children (Ronen & Wozner, 1995; Ronen et al., 1992). Enuretic children were divided into four groups – a waiting-list control group and three treatment groups: token economy, bell-and-pad, and self-control training. All three treatment groups improved as compared with the control group. However, while the rate of success was moderate in the token economy group, the bell-and-pad and self-control training groups exhibited a high rate of success (87%). Furthermore, a major difference appeared between the bell-and-pad and self-control groups regarding a much lower dropout rate for the self-control group and, most significantly, the latter's much lower regression rate at follow-up intervals 3 and 6 months later.

The effectiveness of the model has been demonstrated not only for the treatment of enuresis (Ronen et al., 1992, 1995), but also in single case design studies of the treatment of a young girl suffering from sleep disorders (Ronen, 1993d) and of a young boy with encopresis (Ronen, 1993c). In other studies, the self-control model was found to be very effective in changing 8-year-old children's disobedient behavior at school and 12-year-old children's social problems (Ronen, 1994, 1995). On the basis of this model, Ronen and Rosenbaum (2001) recently developed the SCIM, which aims to impart children both with self-control skills and also with self-help methods to facilitate their future independent functioning. Enhancing children's self-help skills enables them to maintain treatment outcome, continue treating themselves in daily life after successfully being treated by the therapist, generalize and transfer their basic learning, and facilitate self-change.

DESCRIPTION OF THE SELF-CONTROL INTERVENTION MODEL (SCIM)

The SCIM comprises four skill modules, each of which is directed at the teaching of a particular set of self-control skills. Each module is trained under the therapist's full guidance, in two stages: first as general skills and then as related to the specific referred problem. In the first stage, the children initially learn and practice the various skills taught within the four modules, both during the therapy sessions and in homework assignments that offer opportunities for additional exercises and experience. In the second stage, the children are asked to apply each of the four self-control skill modules to the specific problem for which they were referred to therapy. The four SCIM skill modules are presented in Table 5.1.

Cognitive Restructuring

In this skill module, the child is taught that his or her unwanted behavior can be changed, and that like many other kinds of behavior, this change depends on him or her (Beck et al., 1979; Ellis, 1962). Self-efficacy (Bandura, 1997) is a major target at this point in the intervention. Individuals who do not believe in their ability to control themselves have been described as developing helplessness and depression and as maintaining the problems they present (Langer, 1983). To promote a restructuring of the child's maladaptive cognitions, there is a need for redefinition, changing attributional style, and reframing the child's present functioning (Beck et al., 1979; Kanfer & Schefft, 1988; Meichenbaum, 1979). Socratic questions and paradoxical examples can foster the child's understanding that the

Table 5.1. The Four Modules Comprising the Self-Control Intervention Model (SCIM)

Cognitive restructuring	Problem analysis	Attentional focus	Self-control
Redefinition	Linking thoughts & emotions to behaviors	Increasing awareness	Exercising self-talk
Changing attributional style	Linking cause to effect	Identifying internal cues	Self-reward
Reframing		Sensitization	Monitoring
Self-efficacy			Overcoming temptation

problem is a function of motivation and will power, rather than of bad luck or illness. The Socratic method poses questions whose answers are very familiar to the client, in order for the client to be the one who comes up with the answer, inducing him or her to give more thought to the issue.

Problem Analysis

The objective of the second skill module is to help the child understand the process that evolved into the occurrence of the identified problem. Thus, the child is trained to observe the connections between the brain, body, and final problematic behaviors. Focus is placed on teaching the child to notice the links between thoughts, emotions, and behaviors and to learn the link between cause and effect (Beck et al., 1979; Ronen, 1997b). The underlying assumption is that children will find it easier to change their behavior after understanding how their problem behaviors emerged and how they are affected by different thoughts and feelings. Understanding the processes leading up to behavior has been identified as an important variable in improving clients' compliance with and adherence to treatment and also in increasing their efforts to overcome their problems (Meichenbaum & Turk, 1987).

The problem analysis module is administered through rational analysis of these processes, using written materials and anatomical illustrations of the human body, and through helping the child to accept responsibility for the process by learning to change the brain's commands. The child practices identifying automatic thoughts and using self-talk and self-recording to change unmediated thoughts into mediated ones.

Attentional Focus

Here the child is trained to increase awareness of his or her behavior in general, to raise sensitivity to his or her body, and particularly to identify internal cues related to the specific problem (Bandura, 1969, 1997; Mahoney, 1991). Although internal stimuli are difficult to identify, they have as strong an influence on behavior as do external stimuli (Bandura, 1969). Awareness of internal stimuli is an important step towards controlling one's own behavior in that it helps in early identification of sensations, emotions, and behaviors (Bandura, 1969, 1997). Also, being aware of internal stimuli helps in changing unmediated processes into mediated ones (Kanfer & Philips, 1970; Miller, 1979). Relaxation, concentration, and self-monitoring help achieve these targets.

Self-Control Practice

Within the fourth skill module, the child is trained in self-control techniques such as self-talk, self-evaluation, self-monitoring, thinking aloud, and problem solving skills (Barrios & Hartman, 1988; Brigham et al., 1979; Elias et al., 1986; Kendall & Braswell, 1985; Ronen, 1992, 1997b). In the first stage of general skills training, various kinds of practicing are assigned. Practice includes using self-instruction, both in the sessions and in homework assignments to overcome disappointments. Children are asked to exercise self-control in day-to-day activities such as to stop talking when they want to say something, to stop in the middle of playing or crying, or to refrain from drinking when thirsty or from eating when hungry. Children are instructed to continue the physical exercises even when they feel tired or experience some other difficulty. In the second stage, when skills are applied to the child's specific referred problem, self-talk may be emphasized for the child who has a fear of the dark, and imagery may best help the child suffering from social avoidance. Through practice, the child learns that as confidence grows, the chances of success also increase (Bandura, 1997). The self-control techniques taught via this module for changing automatic behaviors to mediated ones include physical as well as emotional exercises such as resisting temptation, self-talk, self-reward, problem solving, and the use of imagery exercises (Meichenbaum, 1979; Ronen, 1997b).

* * *

In sum, this chapter has presented the application of a self-control intervention model for helping children change. To fully institute the process of changing the disturbing behavior, the child is regarded as a scientist whose target is to learn how he or she behaves and how to acquire knowledge in order to change. The role of the therapist is as the child's supervisor, to suggest ways for practicing and learning, and to direct the child in the application of newly learned skills.

Part III of the book will present case studies to illustrate how this intervention model has been used to treat different problem areas typifying children's disorders.

III

Childhood Disorders: Reviews and Case Studies

To further the understanding of the developmental, theoretical, and creative components at the heart of my therapeutic approach, I will now describe seven case studies of children whom I treated in my own clinical practice. Their presenting problems characterize some of the most common disorders encountered by child therapists: selective mutism, anxiety disorder, childhood trauma, enuresis, psychosomatic pain, aggression, and depression.

Each chapter in this part of the book comprises two sections. The first provides a brief literature review about the specific problem and the most common treatments for that disorder. The second describes the clinical process for a single client referred for that disorder, adhering as closely as possible to the actual treatment process. While describing the treatment process, I tried to highlight important steps in the decision making process, which illustrate the guidelines for the different phases of intervention presented in Chapter 4, and I explain the choices I made for each case. To avoid breaking the descriptive flow, I did not stop for theoretical interpretation, but rather tried to highlight techniques taken from my self-control model as described in Chapter 5, and to focus on some of the creative modes implemented that were based on developmental and theoretical considerations.

THE SINGLE CASE DESIGN

The case studies in this part of the book used a single case design to demonstrate the efficacy of intervention. The unique feature of the single case design is its capacity to conduct experimental investigations with one single case, that is, one client, whereby the effect of intervention is evaluated and the manner in which change occurs is of central focus (Kazdin, 1982). The efficacy of the single case design lies in its ability to infer about the intervention's effects by utilizing the client as his or her own control (Kazdin, 1982, 1994a). The primary focus of assessment within this design is on the behavior that is to be changed, which is not always obvious and often depends on one's conceptualization of deviant behavior and personal values regarding the desirability of some behaviors rather than others (Kazdin, 1982, 1994a). The employment of single case designs fixes attention on the process rather than the outcome of intervention, with a focus on how the client is changed step by step through therapy (Ronen, 1991, 1993c,d). This design allows therapists to determine what was really effective in the intervention, when, and how, thus making replication of the treatment process easier to accomplish. The single case design shows the effect of the intervention by comparing different conditions or treatment techniques with the same client, trying to pinpoint the changes that occurred (Kazdin, 1994a).

Assessment of performance in single case designs utilizes many procedures and measurements. The main methods comprise assessment of behavior via direct observation of overt performance or via the client's self-report, and comparing changes in those behaviors.

In this part of the book, I will describe different methods for single case design, to suit the specific interventions I will present.

Early Childhood

6

Selective Mutism

LITERATURE REVIEW

Selective mutism was first mentioned in the 19th century by Kussmaul (1877), who described a disorder in which people would not speak in some situations, despite having the ability to speak. Tramer (1934) labeled the disorder elective mutism, with the belief that these children were "electing" not to speak.

Selective mutism comprises a rare psychiatric disorder characterized by the total lack of speech in at least one specific situation (usually the classroom), despite the ability to speak in other situations (Dow et al., 1995; Salvatore et al., 1999). Usually, normal language development is present, but speech occurs only in small groups of relatives and peers (Powell & Dalley, 1995). Children who have this disorder refuse to speak in most social situations, although they may communicate via gestures, head shakes, or monosyllabic words (Jacobson, 1995). The children tend to appear normal and do not usually exhibit the presence of mental or physical defects. Selective mutism may be the manifestation of a shy, inhibited temperament associated with developmental delays, speech and language disabilities, or difficulties in processing social cues (Dow et al., 1995; Salvatore et al., 1999). Often, selective mutism demonstrates comorbidity with other disorders, especially internalizing behavior problems. The most common include anxiety disorders, obsessive-compulsive rituals, social phobia, and depression (Kristensen, 2000; Thomsen et al., 1999). Kristensen assessed the comorbidity of developmental delay in children with selective mutism. Results showed that 68.5% met the criteria for a diagnosis reflecting a developmental disorder. In addition, 74.1% met the criteria for anxiety disorder, and others met criteria for elimination disorders (enuresis, encopresis).

Children suffering from this disorder encompass a heterogeneous group comprising less than 1% of the school-aged population. The disorder is more prevalent in females than males. Parents usually report that the child "has always been this way" (Dow et al., 1995), but the diagnosis is most often not made before the child enters kindergarten or school. The disorder typically starts in early childhood and lasts at least for several months (Jacobson, 1995).

A variety of explanations have been proposed for selective mutism. The disorder has been viewed mainly as a medical problem, and a range of different psychological explanations have been offered relating the disorder to internal psychological conflicts, familial problems, or learning difficulties. These alternative explanations led to various treatments, including the pharmacological, psychodynamic, family, and cognitive and behavioral approaches.

Pharmacotherapy

The medical approach views selective mutism as a medical abnormality. Salvatore and colleagues (1999) showed a deletion of chromosome 18 among children suffering from selective mutism. They claimed that selective mutism appears as a chronic disorder and may be related to a genetic background. They also concluded that a relation exists between selective mutism, the deletion of the short arm of chromosome 12, and the lack of chromosome 18, and they believe this relates to developmental disorders and dysmorphisms. Another orientation (Crumley, 1990) views selective mutism as a genetic characteristic related to a biologically mediated temperament.

The medical treatment of selective mutism is based on different medications to change the child's speaking habits, and is directed toward the child's fears, anxiety, depression, and temperament. Often, pharmacotherapy is administered as part of the psychological treatment process.

Thomsen and colleagues (1999) described a successful treatment of a 17-year-old girl with selective mutism, using Citalopram. This girl had a long history of treatment, including family therapy, individual psychotherapy, individual behavior therapy, and milieu therapy. None of these treatments had resulted in any significant improvement. In the present treatment, they prescribed Citalopram, a highly specific serotonin reuptake inhibitor with a maximum dosage of 40 mg per day. They reported good results without side effects.

Another case study presented the efficacy and acceptability of Sertaline treatment in eliminating mutism among 5–17-year-old children (Carlson et al., 1999). Rupp (1999) presented a case study of treatment for a 5-year-old girl with selective mutism, using Haloperidol, which is usually prescribed for children suffering from Tourette's disorder, and showed its effectiveness in reducing her selective mutism behavior.

Psychodynamic Therapy

The psychodynamic approach views selective mutism as a manifestation of intrapsychic conflict, a neurosis, or a symptom reflecting an unresolved psychodynamic conflict (Youngerman, 1979). This conflict is usually characterized by overprotective or domineering mothers and strict or remote fathers (Dow et al., 1995).

Psychodynamic therapy focuses on identifying and resolving such underlying conflicts. Jacobson (1995) described one four-year treatment of a client; however, not many other descriptions or studies are available on its application.

Family Therapy

The family approach views the disorder as a result of interactions within the family, but, again, no systematic research has been conducted on treatment procedures. Robin (1999) suggested that selective mutism stems from dysfunction with the family system, especially a mother who tends to be enmeshed with the child, and a father who is frequently disengaged from the family. She proposed that the entire family system be treated using a collaborative multimodal approach. Robin pointed out the importance of therapeutic relationships in successfully treating selective mutism.

Cognitive and Behavioral Therapies

The cognitive behavioral approach views selective mutism as a personal response to trauma. For example, children might be reacting to a trauma such as sexual abuse, early hospitalization, divorce, or death (MacGregor et al., 1994). Some view the disorder as a kind of social phobia (Black & Ude, 1992; Jacobson, 1995). Others explain it as the desire for control, a manipulation of the environment by the child who wishes to control others as well as the wish to control his or her own anxiety (Powell & Dalley, 1995).

Cognitive behavioral therapy is the most common treatment for this disorder, in addition to pharmacotherapy, particularly behavioral interventions based on principles of learning theory. Redd (1963) was the first to suggest the application of reinforcement and stimulus fading under the hypothesis that mutism developed either as a means of getting attention or as an escape from anxiety. Treatments target the extinguishing of all reinforcement for the mutism, while simultaneously bolstering self-confidence and decreasing anxiety. Other modalities combine positive reinforcement, shaping, desensitization, modeling, and extinction (Powell & Dalley, 1995). Descriptions are available of shaping speech by reinforcing mouth movements that proximate speech until true speech is achieved, and of self-modeling, where children watch videotaped segments of themselves performing desired behaviors (Dow et al., 1995). It is recommended that the child not be forced to speak, but rather should be offered behavioral play therapy to reinforce speech, so that this nonverbal disorder will receive a nonverbal solution (Powell & Dalley, 1995). Mark and Douglas (1999) described a long-term therapy for a seventh grade boy who had selective mutism since kindergarten. The treatment consisted of systematic desensitization, consultation with school personnel, and training in social speaking skills.

Lack of research, difficulties in assessment, and the lack of clearly effective treatments characterize the selective mutism disorder. Problems in researching this area relate to the fact that most of the documentation on selective mutism is based on single-case studies. Black and Ude (1992), for example, described a girl who had told her mother she was reluctant to speak because her voice sounded strange and she did not want others to hear it. Zelenko and Shaw (2000) presented the treatment of a 7-year-old Mexican boy in the U.S., and they attributed his disorder to the unique nature of immigrant families.

Assessment of selective mutism is difficult, in that most of these children will not speak to therapists and must be assessed through parents or teachers. Information is collected on the child's ability to speak, the people with whom he or she does speak, the degree to which the child is verbally and nonverbally inhibited, academic abilities, and other disorders or symptoms. Interviewing the child is difficult, although necessary, and focuses on direct observation of temperament, quality of interaction, and the ability to communicate verbally and nonverbally. Assessment is conducted through nonverbal communication modes such as playing and drawing.

Problems in the treatment of selective mutism relate to the severity of the disorder and to the paucity of research on treatment efficacy. Treatment for selective mutism has long been considered difficult by all therapeutic approaches, with some even describing it as "intractable" (Dow et al., 1995).

The following case study describes a creative self-control treatment with a young boy suffering from selective mutism.

BEN'S STORY OF SILENCE

Assessing Ben's Behavior

First intake session. Ben was almost 6 years old when I first met him. He was brought to me during his last months of kindergarten, about four months before he was to enter the first grade in school. The reason for referral was selective mutism. As I met with Ben and his parents, I could not ignore his big brown eyes and the intelligent, smiling look I saw in them whenever I gave an interpretation of his situation.

As mentioned in Part II, we start assessing the client and the family from the minute they enter the room. The fact that Ben did not talk made me focus on his nonverbal communication. A very important role in my assessment of Ben was played by his physical behavior and facial expressions: the way he sat, the movement of his face, his body language, etc.

For the purpose of accurate diagnosis, I also needed some other assessment tools. As outlined in Chapter 4, in order to select reliable and valid assessment tools for assessing Ben, I had to relate to his age (see Table 4.3) and to the nature of his problem, the mutism behavior, which suggested the need for removing his anxiety and increasing his social behavior (see Table 4.2). At $5\frac{1}{2}$ years of age, Ben was in the stage of early childhood. At this stage, children's disorders usually relate to the ability to master social and academic situations, and parental discipline. Assessment of children at that age, therefore, is based on environmental reports, in this case from the parents, his kindergarten teacher, and a physical therapist working with Ben on motor problems. In terms of the problem type, it is strongly recommended that assessment of overcontrolled disorders like Ben's be solidly based on the most reliable source of information: self-reports and emotional questionnaires administered to Ben himself. However, the fact that Ben did not talk precluded the usage of such tools, providing another reason to decide to focus assessment on environmental reports. In particular, his age and behavior warranted a direct observation of his conduct at the kindergarten. All of these assessment methods contributed to my conclusions about Ben's behavior and served as baseline data for later evaluation of his progress.

Parents' report. During the intake session, the parents reported that the only people with whom Ben talked were themselves and his 4-year-old sister. He had never talked with anyone else. Because of Ben's father's work, the family had been traveling around the world, and they had just returned from a three-year stay in a country where a different language was spoken. Ben attended kindergarten there, but never talked. His mother reported that he had been in dynamic play therapy there for the last two years, but he had refused to talk even with the therapist. They remembered him beginning to talk as a baby, but soon enough, right after moving overseas, he started to get along by pointing at things and not talking. In the presence of others, he would whisper in his parents' ears, but no one else had ever heard his voice. They were worried how he would get along in school and therefore came to me for therapy.

Kindergarten teacher's report. Following the intake session, after receiving the parents' agreement, I went to visit the kindergarten with a dual purpose in mind: to interview the kindergarten teacher and to directly observe Ben's behavior. The teacher reported that Ben was very active and participated in all activities, but without talking. He would point at the things he wanted, use hand gestures, and make strange facial expressions, which would generally make him the center of attention. When he did not receive what he wanted, he used to cry and shout. As a result, the staff as well as the other children were constantly busy trying to satisfy Ben's needs and prevent his outbursts. The teacher reported him to be a very difficult child to handle. She was highly interested in getting Ben to talk and had attempted many times to persuade him to speak with her.

Direct observation in the kindergarten. In my observations of Ben's behavior while playing outside on the kindergarten playground, I was impressed by the way in which he was able to acquire whatever he wanted without talking. He pointed at things, and, amazingly, all the children were very enthusiastic to get him what he wanted. My impression was that Ben played a very central role among his classmates, who competed with each other as to who would best understand Ben's gestures and who would be the first to bring him what he desired.

Physical therapist's report. Ben was in physical therapy due to some fine motor problems, and I asked for the parents' permission to speak with his physiotherapist. I was impressed that here, again, Ben was able to focus attention on his incapacity to speak and was able to obtain whatever he wanted without the need to talk. The physiotherapist, like the kindergarten teacher, was eager to be the one who would make him start talking. Throughout her sessions, she also invested efforts in persuading him and trying to trick him to talk.

Baseline Data: Drawing Conclusions from the Assessment

Assessment of Ben was based on the first intake session with Ben and his parents, the kindergarten teacher's and physical therapist's reports, and my direct observation of Ben. All these sources of information pointed to the fact that Ben did not talk, not even a word, and that Ben was able to get along without talking. Altogether, the assessment process with Ben, his family, and his environment led me to raise several assumptions:

1. The parents reported his speech at home to be normal, and both they and the kindergarten teacher reported that Ben seemed to be very intelligent. His lack of speech, therefore, did not appear to be related either to language deficiencies or to intellectual or developmental problems.
2. Ben had the ability to talk, and he seemed to be manipulating the environment by not talking. It was a matter of power, not a matter of weakness or lack of power. In other words, Ben was trying to control his surroundings and seemed to have developed a way of obtaining whatever he wanted. His ability to communicate without talking seemed to further increase his avoidance behavior, which only increased the anxiety he felt, in turn making it even more difficult for him to start talking. I believed that the longer he managed without talking, the more difficult it would be for him to start talking again.
3. Ben was introduced to everyone by his parents (including to me) as a very smart boy. His parents emphasized that he could read, write, and understand everything. I assumed that this introduction increased Ben's anxiety and his fear of disappointing the environment if he started talking and people saw he was not as smart as they thought he was.

4. Ben intentionally focused attention on his inability to talk. By not talking, Ben received a great deal of attention. People were forced to look carefully at him to identify his signals, and they often tried to help him. I had a strong feeling that Ben's behavior had been reinforced by the whole neighborhood, and he would be very reluctant to give up these secondary gains.

In order to make the decision as to whether or not Ben's behavior was deviant and necessitated intervention, who in his environment should be treated, and how, I followed the different phases described in Chapter 4.

Phase 1 of Decision Making: Does Ben Need Therapy or Not?

The first phase of intervention with Ben required a decision as to whether or not his presented behavior warranted therapy. As described in Chapter 4, four main variables contributed to making this decision: problem variables, developmental and environmental variables, child and family variables, and treatment variables.

With regard to problem variables, Ben's mutism behavior was examined in terms of the *DSM-IV* diagnostic criteria (American Psychiatric Association, 1994) and was found to correspond to the diagnosis of selective mutism. Ben had refrained from talking for longer than six months. His behavior had not improved, and the chances for spontaneous recovery were low. At his age, children are still developing their language skills. They also start developing social relationships, and those linguistic and interpersonal skills are very important for further development. Not being able to talk with peers might pose a risk to Ben's ability to grow up as a self-confident child who could express his needs and adapt well to his social environment, thus suggesting a high risk for his future.

A comparison of Ben's behavior to social developmental norms highlighted his deviance from peers his age, who talked fluently. His behavior also deviated from his sex group and cultural group. Moreover, the family members viewed his behavior as very abnormal.

In terms of child and family variables, the parents evidenced great motivation for change. They were ready to comply with the treatment, seemed extremely supportive, and really wanted Ben to overcome his problems. The parents were very upset by Ben's behavior and were afraid for his future. They expressed willingness to adhere to every instruction in order to help him start talking. The kindergarten teacher could also serve as a support system, as well as could the peers who seemed to care for him. On the other hand, Ben himself was not enthusiastic for change and initially did not seem to want to comply with therapy. I believed that his reluctance stemmed from his fear of change, fear that he would no longer be able to acquire whatever he wanted, and fear of losing the attention to which he had grown accustomed. I thought I could secure his agreement to cooperate if I were careful not to push him to start talking, and at the same time if I showed him that he could gain much more attention if he were to talk. I was therefore not disturbed by his unwillingness to cooperate; I viewed it as his preliminary stage of testing me and what I had to offer through treatment.

Referring to treatment variables, selective mutism is a disorder that has good prognostic chances. There was no reason to expect spontaneous recovery because Ben's condition had only deteriorated. The most problematic issue to consider was how to develop a good therapeutic relationship, in light of Ben's resistance and refusal to talk. This issue will be addressed later on.

Thus, the first phase of the decision making process clearly indicated that Ben should receive treatment as soon as possible in order to cease his speech avoidance and to prevent future damage to his healthy social and emotional development.

Phase 2 of Decision Making: Classifying Ben's Referral and Goals for Change

The second phase of decision making involved assessing Ben's referral and establishing treatment goals in terms of the therapeutic goals and developmental tasks outlined in Chapter 4. In relation to referral goals, out of the four reasons for referral of children's disorders, two were very important for Ben. The first comprised removing the anxiety that caused his avoidance behavior. Plainly, Ben suffered from anxiety that prevented him from trying to talk. He was afraid of losing attention, of revealing himself to be less intelligent than people thought he was, and of being unable to comply with other's wishes. The need to remove anxiety was therefore extremely crucial for him. Also, Ben lacked appropriate, mature social skills that could assist him in acquiring self-confidence and self-trust. Increasing his social behavior, in terms of the ability to establish and maintain contact with others, therefore constituted another important goal of therapy. These two goals coincide with overcontrolled behaviors, which characterize children who are afraid to let go of control due to their high expectations, exaggerated self-criteria for achievement, and constant need for others' approval. Thus, these two goals were identified as the main issues to address in therapy.

Relating to developmental stages, Ben, at the end of early childhood, was about to enter school. This is a stage where the social tasks revolve around mastering academic and social skills. Ben would need to learn to master academic assignments, especially those involving the use of language. The ability to speak would become far more crucial as he entered school, and therefore it was determined that removing his anxiety and increasing his ability to speak should be at the center of treatment.

Phase 3 of Decision Making: Selecting Who Should Be Treated

In considering who should be treated, I decided to supervise Ben's environmental settings, to counsel his parents, and to treat Ben directly in the presence of his parents. These decisions were based on developmental considerations and on the nature of Ben's referred problem. Usually at this age, it is easier to supervise the environment than to treat the child (see Table 4.4). Intervention in Ben's environment was also indicated by the nature of his problem, in order to eliminate the strong reinforcement of his behavior by his parents and kindergarten environment, diminish the stress of their high expectations and demands, and remove the secondary effects of his silence (i.e. the attention). The nature of Ben's disorder (overcontrolled behavior), involving anxiety and fears, also indicated the need to directly treat Ben (see Table 4.5). Individual treatment would focus on increasing his self-confidence and self-efficacy; introducing exposure assignments to stop his avoidance behaviors; and reinforcing the positive behavior of talking. Treatment thus involved counseling the parents, kindergarten teacher, and physical therapist, as well as individual therapy with Ben.

Phase 4 of Decision Making: Selecting Ben's Optimal Treatment Modes

In determining the specific treatment methods, it seemed that supervision of Ben's environment could easily be conducted verbally, based on cognitive behavior methods. It appeared more difficult to design treatment techniques and methods to directly treat Ben. Usually at Ben's age (early childhood), the treatment of choice is nonverbal therapy. Preschool children typically evidence difficulties in focusing attention, limited language skills, and immature ways of thinking. Therefore, nonverbal methods are often applicable such as drawing, movement, music, or play methods (see Table 4.6). However, individual differences, namely, Ben's mature behavior and above-age comprehension level, indicated that he would have been a good candidate for verbal therapy if he had been ready to talk. Nevertheless, the kind of disorder Ben (evidenced selective mutism) clearly indicated the need to apply nonverbal treatment methods that would not pressure him to talk when he refused. Hence, I decided to design a treatment method that would combine verbal therapy (mostly from my side, that is, I would do the talking) with nonverbal methods, primarily the creative techniques of drawing and playing.

Counseling and Supervising the Environment

As a first stage, it seemed important to supervise the kindergarten in how to deal with Ben. As I described above, Ben was in the habit of pointing or gesturing with his hands or head, and the other children, who liked him, were accustomed to watching him carefully and helping him if they could. Everyone in the kindergarten needed instruction in how to stop placing Ben at the center of attention and how to stop "helping" him in the form of talking in his stead or bringing him whatever he indicated. The staff was instructed to refrain from giving Ben objects, and to stop verbalizing for him. They were also asked to act as if they did not understand his hints and gestures. In that way, his silence would become problematic for him. However, it was very difficult to implement a change among the children. As mentioned before, they competed and challenged each other to see who would be the first to fulfill his silent requests and "who had ever heard Ben talking." I asked the kindergarten teacher to talk with the children (when Ben was not present). She was instructed to tell them that everyone has difficulties of some kind or another. Being a good friend to Ben meant that they could help him by not discussing with him his ability to speak. Instead, they were asked to try and play with him naturally.

The physical therapist was instructed to stop trying to make him talk and to concentrate on her work. She was also asked to act as if she did not understand his hints, in order to reduce the efficacy of his nonverbal substitutes for oral communication.

The parents were instructed to stop lecturing Ben about how important it was for him to talk. They had to stop discussing his behavior in front of him at all. In fact, they were asked to stop helping him. For example, if he wanted food at a restaurant, his parents were not to speak for him but rather were to ask him to tell the waiter what to bring him. (At this point, Ben masterfully continued to manage without speech, by pointing at the menu until the waiter understood.) Or, his mother was instructed to stop calling and asking friends over for Ben. She was advised to tell him, "If you want to invite a friend, you are welcome to do so." It became his responsibility to invite friends over by himself if he wanted. When he complained of headaches, he was now told to talk directly with the physician. He had to explain the problem himself, without his mother as the intermediary.

Individual Treatment of Ben

The first individual session was aimed toward creating an alliance with Ben. I was hoping to gain an understanding of how he felt about his problem, and to obtain his agreement and collaboration for change. I told Ben it was very important for me to understand him in order to help him. I said I would talk with him but that he did not have to answer verbally; he could find any other way he wished to communicate his ideas.

During this first session, I asked Ben to draw the way he felt. He drew a picture of a ball rolling and rolling. When I asked Ben what he meant, he started jumping and rolling around the room as if to show me that he could not control his behavior any longer. Then, he took a piece of paper, drew all kinds of lines, and wrote: "one big mess." Ben felt his life was one big mess going out of control, and he did not know how to deal with it.

Ben agreed nonverbally that he was ready to work with me, and we decided to start therapy. For the next six sessions, as he entered the room each time, he immediately took out a box of plastic building blocks. He would then dump them all out and then try to throw and break them. While doing this, he would look at me to see how I would respond. Each time, I took the blocks, put them aside, and said, "Sorry. You're welcome to play with them if you ask for them and take good care of them, but here you are not going to break them." It seemed as if Ben was trying to control the world through his behavior. With me, his lack of speech was not a problem, so he tried to find other ways to test and control me. Gradually, he started a new stage of entering the room, looking at me, smiling, and pointing at the box of blocks. Later on, when asking for the blocks, he even exaggeratedly bowed down while making the gesture of "please" and smiling at me. I felt that this initial setting of limits had relieved Ben somewhat of the urge to try to control me with his silence. He had learned that therapy held a different set of rules, where he could be himself more, relax a bit, and channel his efforts into starting to learn and to change his behavior.

Clarifying the purposes and plan of therapy. I used to talk with Ben's parents at the end of each session. They told me how he used to return from physical therapy or his previous psychotherapy and would mock those therapists' interpretation of Ben as a weak, poor, suffering child. He rebelled against the idea that "other people think they know what I feel better than I do." It was important for me to let Ben feel that I was there for him, to help him understand his life and his problem, and not to force my own interpretations on him.

I realized that the basic constructivist notion of "meaning making process" (Mahoney, 1991) could be of great importance for collaboration with Ben. I told him that I wished to understand him better but would need his help, and only then would we be able to establish criteria and aims for treatment. Showing him the picture he drew earlier of a mess, I gave Ben a ball of yarn, asking him if he could show me the way he felt, that mess, using the yarn. He took the ball, unraveled all the wool, and then tied it up into a knotted snarl! I said, "Well, it is a big mess. Would you like us to work together in trying to untangle it and set it down so that it will become one long, straight strand of wool?" He looked at me, took the yarn, tried to open the knot, and tore it. I said, "Well, it's not going to be easy; we'll need time and patience. But if you have these, so do I. Whenever you get tired of working on it, either we'll rest or I'll take your place. What do you think?" Ben looked at me, waited for a while, and then nodded "yes" with his head. I asked him who he thought could help in putting things in order, and he wrote: "parents, friends, me, you."

I asked Ben if I could summarize our agreement as a contract. He assented, and I wrote it down (see Figure 6.1).

After signing the agreement, Ben added in writing: "The agreement is with Tammie, not with my parents, and the meetings are with Tammie, not with my parents."

Ben describes his life as one big mess, like a ball of wool with many knots. The purpose of our meeting, therefore, is to organize the knots and put things back in order. As a therapist, my role is to try and understand Ben, to propose ways to help him change, and to practice these ways with him.

Ben's role is to listen to Tammie's suggestions, correct her if she is mistaken, help her understand him better, and cooperate in practicing.

We thereby agree that every method and technique will be mutually decided upon and that together we will measure Ben's progress.

Signatures: ____________________

____

Figure 6.1. Agreement between Ben and Tammie.

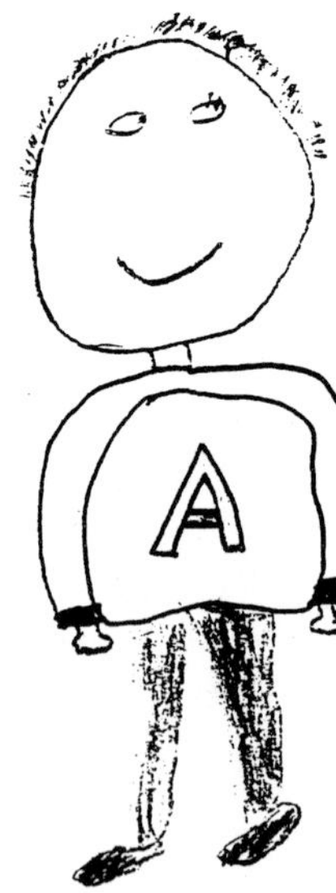

Figure 6.2 Ben's drawing of himself from the outside.

Ben's mother later told me that after this meeting he was very satisfied, saying: "Tammie isn't going to treat me. We're going to study and practice together. She'll tell me and I'll tell her."

The next time that I asked Ben to draw himself, he drew a very large boy (see Figure 6.2), and immediately afterwards drew a picture of a very small boy (see Figure 6.3). When I asked about the two, he wrote on the larger boy: "Me from the outside, what others see." On the small boy's picture he wrote: "Me from the inside, what I see." Ben's wonderful ability to express himself by reading and

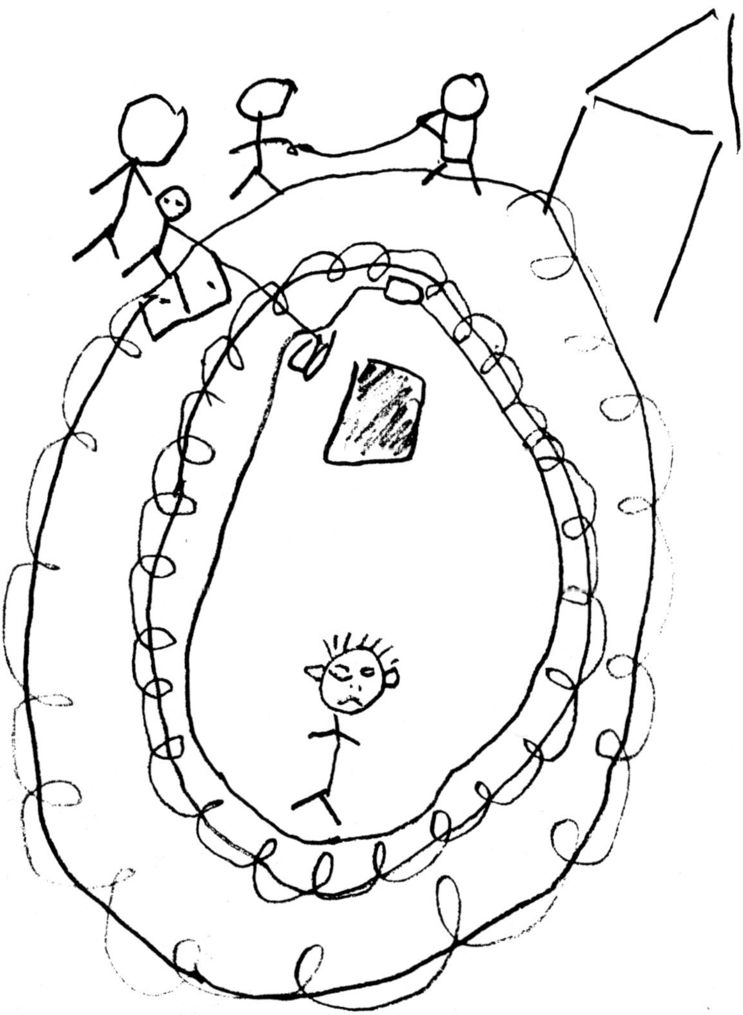

Figure 6.3. Ben's drawing of himself from the inside.

writing, developed at a very young age, had helped him to cope with his selective mutism and now was facilitating his expression in therapy. I used his expressiveness to establish another treatment goal: "You know, by untying the yarn and arranging the mess, we will try to make the inside of you look and feel the same as the outside of you." Ben was happy and agreed to work toward that purpose. As we continued to work together, I based Ben's treatment on my self-control intervention model (SCIM; see Table 5.1), which I translated to nonverbal, creative methods in order to demonstrate the needed phases.

SCIM module 1: Cognitive restructuring and redefinition. In the next session, I told Ben that untying the yarn would necessitate a lot of control and, therefore, I would like to impart him with the necessary skills to control himself. One purpose of this session was to modify Ben's attributional style by teaching him that selective mutism was a behavior that, for different reasons, he himself had chosen to perform. I said that changing a behavior that one picked oneself is very difficult, but that it was up to him to do so. I told him that I believed that when he felt confident enough, he would be able to do it. During that session, I tried to redefine Ben's behavior as "the preference not to talk" rather than "the inability to talk." Up until this time, Ben believed he was " incapable of talking due to his fears." I redefined his behavior as "feeling afraid of taking the risk of talking." Using the first module of the intervention, I wanted Ben to reconstruct his thoughts and gain a new self-efficacy, thus relating the disorder to his wishes and his goals.

I knew it was hard for Ben to change. I also knew that the more he had been asked to change, the more difficult it had become for him to do so. At that stage, I only wanted him to start questioning whether or not it was his own decision, whether he could change it himself, and whether or not it was worth the effort.

SCIM module 2: Problem analysis. At this stage in the intervention process, I wished to help Ben link his thoughts to emotions and behaviors and to learn about causes and effects. I tried to analyze his lack of speech as a command issued from his brain, which resulted from his fears.

In trying to understand his reasons for not talking, I suggested some ideas in writing, such as: "I'm afraid to sound foolish," "My language isn't good enough," and "No one will pay attention to me." I proposed that such thoughts and feelings might result in his mute behavior. Ben reacted with anger toward me, tore up the paper, and wrote: "You're stupid. I can't talk. I'm not big enough." Yet I felt it important not to abandon this issue, so I slowly continued talking about it. He felt better when I added that I did not mean for him to start talking immediately. I only wanted him to understand the way his silence worked. To understand why things happened, so that sometime in the future, not now, but later, when he felt confident enough, he would be able to choose to start talking. In order to make it easier for him to understand, we drew a table (see Table 6.1).

Table 6.1. The Links Between Ben's Thoughts, Emotions, and Behaviors

Event	Automatic thought	Emotion	Behavior
Kids are gathering around me	I won't know what to say to them	Afraid, tense	Avoid talking
The kindergarten teacher asks me a question	What if I don't know the answer?	Anxious, nervous	Refrain from speaking

Table 6.2. Ben's Other-Related Examples of the Link Between Cognitions, Affects, and Behaviors

Thought	Emotion	Behavior
They're trying to force me to talk	I hate to be forced	I behave stubbornly
All the children are interested in me this way	I'm afraid they won't be interested any longer if I talk	I keep silent

This technique was first offered by Beck et al. (1979) as a means to help clients change their negative automatic thoughts into positive mediated ones. Ronen and Rosenbaum (1998) adapted the technique to enhance the understanding of the client's general meaning-making processes. The technique focuses on the person's cognition (verbal or pictorial "events" in the stream of consciousness) in an attempt to link thoughts and emotions to behaviors (Beck, 1963). Thus, new learning experiences are designed that remedy the dysfunctional or distorted cognitions, behaviors, and affective patterns (Kendall & Braswell, 1985).

Ben was willing to listen to this line of thinking, and he even found it amusing to try to guess his own thoughts and behaviors. Through this table, Ben learned that whatever happened to him had an interpretation, an automatic thought that gave meaning to the situation in his eyes. Usually, the meaning was negative, such as: "I'm going to fail," "I can't do it," or "They'll laugh at me." These negative thoughts elicited the stressful, fearful emotions that caused him not to talk. It was important for me that Ben realize that avoidance of talking was not a sickness or a deficiency but rather a behavior he himself had chosen.

As happened with Ben often, once he cooperated with this table-making exercise and understood the principle, he turned things around to serve a different purpose of his own. Instead of using such a table to understand how the brain commanded him not to speak, he designed another, similar table to explain how others made him feel uncomfortable (see Table 6.2).

We discussed Ben's feeling while being forced, while being afraid of something, and I used his examples to focus on how important it is for him, to learn to control himself rather than being controlled by others.

SCIM module 3: Attentional focus. In this module, Ben was taught to identify his internal cues and to become aware of his feelings, sensations, and emotions. Ben was very impulsive in his behavior, and he usually acted (e.g. crying, shouting, throwing objects) before having the time to evaluate his own feelings in different situations. I believed part of his problem was related to his inability to understand and identify the anxiety, fear, shyness, as well as the happiness he felt.

Ben was asked to keep a chart of his feelings over the next three weeks. He was asked to note every day how happy, sad, or fearful he was in kindergarten, along a scale of 0–10 (see Table 6.3). He was also asked to record where in his own body he had those sensations (e.g. chest, face, throat) and to describe the type and strength of the sensations (e.g. shooting pain, butterflies, warm flush). In order to tangibly explain the meaning of the numerical scale to Ben, I brought a ladder into the room. I used it to demonstrate how each rung was higher than the one below, just as people can feel increasing emotional intensity, for example, from slightly happy (0) to extremely happy (10). Ben initially refused to admit that he ever felt anxious or fearful, but he took the chart home and agreed to keep a record.

Ben returned to the following session with an empty chart. He wrote to me that I had given him a stupid assignment. I told him that he made me sad, because it would now be more difficult for me to teach him how to overcome the emotions he did not like. As I spoke, Ben moved closer to me. I then explained how important it was to identify emotions in order to become able to control and change them. He liked the idea of control, and the next week he arrived with a completed chart (see Table 6.4).

Table 6.3. Suggested Chart Assigned to Ben: Emotions' Extent, Location, and Type

Today I felt	(little → lot)	Where I felt it	What I felt
Happy	0 1 2 3 4 5 6 7 8 9 10		
Sad	0 1 2 3 4 5 6 7 8 9 10		
Excited	0 1 2 3 4 5 6 7 8 9 10		
Angry	0 1 2 3 4 5 6 7 8 9 10		
Fearful	0 1 2 3 4 5 6 7 8 9 10		

Table 6.4. Ben's First Weekly Chart of Emotions

Today in kindergarten I felt	Scale	Where I felt it	What I felt
Bored	10	In my eyes	They were closing
Tired	10	All my body	Wanted to sleep
Angry	9	My mouth	Wanted to kill my kindergarten teacher

With me speaking and Ben responding in writing, we discussed the emotions he had recorded and the ways children usually express them. I told him I was sad because most of the time he had negative emotions. I said I could understand that he was angry, sad, and tired, but I also wished for him to feel happy and excited. Two more weeks passed before Ben was able to write down that he was happy during a birthday party in the kindergarten and when his father gave him a present, and that he was excited when his grandparents came to visit. At this stage, we could begin talking differentially about his emotions and about what he felt toward various people and in diverse situations.

SCIM module 4: Self-control exercises. The next aim of treatment consisted of imparting self-control techniques to change Ben's behavior, increase his confidence, and gradually enable him to talk. I felt paradoxical interventions suited Ben because of his tendency to enter power struggles and to demonstrate resistance to adults' pressures or demands. This technique neutralized Ben's struggle by giving him a challenge in the direction opposite to the true objective, and allowing him to believe he was still resisting.

I offered him an exercise in the form of a challenge: "Just make sure you don't forget how to talk! Why don't you pick a different person every day and say something silly to them?" Ben accepted the challenge, and he chose to talk to a stranger in the street, his pediatrician, and his dentist, but he would not talk with friends or relatives. I was very careful not to ask him to talk with me. I emphasized the fact that he did not have to talk to me, but that maybe he should consider doing so, just to make sure he still remembered how. I also commented that, if and when he did decide to talk to me, he better do it when no one else could hear, so that people would not think he had already resolved his problem.

Another part of the self-control exercise module comprised learning to use problem-solving methods, and especially learning to evaluate and predict outcomes and cost-effect considerations. I asked Ben to think of all the benefits he gained from not talking, and he made a list of advantages:

Advantages
I can annoy my parents
The kids watch me
I don't have to do what they want
People don't shout at me
I do whatever I want

I asked him to make another list, of disadvantages, but he refused. I then wrote such a list myself while he watched me:

Disadvantages
I don't have friends
I can't take part in discussions at kindergarten
People think I'm stupid, they don't know I'm smart

I can't tell them if I'm happy or sad
I can't argue and win an argument
I'm becoming more and more frightened
Life isn't fun

Ben became angry with me, tore up the paper, pushed me, and left the room. Then, he came back, yelled, and left the room again. I said, "I know you're angry, and you probably have the right to be angry. But, I am sorry you can not express your emotion instead of behaving the way you do".

To the next session, Ben arrived with a picture of a human body, and on its head he wrote, "You have a stupid brain. You don't understand. I cannot talk." I asked him what he *could* do, and he replied, "I can write, draw, and cry." At the entrance to the clinic, he saw the ladder and gestured, "Why is it there?" I told him we could use it if he wanted. I then took two pieces of paper. On the first I wrote: "Being able to control myself. Being able to talk when I wish and to be quiet when I wish." I taped this to the top rung of the ladder. On the second paper, which I placed on the bottom rung, I wrote: "Others control me. I can't talk as I wish."

Ben looked at me, took some paper, and wrote: "I can talk when I wish but I'm afraid." I told Ben I thought that his words showed great progress and that, by admitting he was afraid to talk, he had really begun to unravel the mess. I took his hand and asked him to climb the first rung of the ladder. I then asked him: "How do you feel to be on the first rung and not on the floor?" He pointed at the top rung and, for the first time, moved his lips as if talking, although no voice came out. He mouthed: "I want to be up there." I replied, "No, it's too early and that's too high. I'm afraid to go so fast because you might fall. You have to decide very carefully if and when you wish to talk."

Our goal for that week was that Ben would call and invite a friend over by himself. He did so, and in the next session he reported that all the children had surrounded him the next day, imploring "We also want to hear if you can talk." There was no way to prevent this; however, I told Ben he should not be afraid of changing, because the children would be even more interested with him if he started talking. Ben looked at me suspiciously, but his mother told me that in the following weeks he was continuing to invite friends over. It seemed as if at that time he was struggling. He was still afraid, and he still would not talk to me, but he had begun to understand the benefits of talking and had begun to doubt whether he should continue to refrain from talking. I could see the change in his beliefs; he stopped arguing about whether or not he could in fact talk, and he was ready to admit that he could talk but was afraid to.

The summer vacation was approaching and, in consultation with his parents, I recommended sending Ben to swimming classes in another city, so that he would not meet children he knew. I also occasionally mentioned to him: "You know that they don't know you can't talk, and it's very dangerous not to talk while swimming, because you won't be able to let them know if you're in trouble in the water."

The next week, as Ben entered the room, he spoke aloud to me for the first time, saying loudly: "I talked!" I was very excited but pretended I hadn't noticed and replied, "I don't understand. What do you mean? Write it to me!" He again shouted, "I talked!" and then wrote down: "No one in swimming knows I can't talk. I talked with them."

The parents also followed my suggestion to send Ben to a summer day camp, again far from home. Together with Ben, I redefined his problem: "I can talk easily, and it's not a problem to talk with people who don't know me. What's hard is to start talking with people who already know me as someone who can't talk."

Ben agreed with this new definition. I added a blank piece of paper to the second rung of the ladder, inviting Ben to label it. He climbed to the second rung and wrote on the paper, "Higher is nicer." We then discussed, with Ben still writing, his ability to climb up and progress and the way he was doing it. I redefined his behavior, not as he said "I'm weak and afraid," but as, "You're strong and brave, and it's not easy to make changes, but you can and you did. I'm very proud and you can be very satisfied with yourself."

Ben then asked me if I wanted him to talk with me, and then wrote: "But you know me as not talking." I answered, "Well, would you like to pretend it isn't me?" We started role playing. I was Diane, the counselor at camp, and he was the talking Ben. For the next few sessions, as he arrived, he would tell me who I was to be and what kind of communication we were going to have. If I was Tammie, it meant that we were going to talk about his problems, using nonverbal techniques. If I was someone else, we could talk fluently.

From this point on, Ben progressed very quickly, and in a month, he was talking with everyone except his physiotherapist. In fact, his parents claimed he was talking too much.

Phase 5 of Decision Making: Evaluating Ben at the End of Therapy and Maintaining Treatment Outcomes

Evaluation. As mentioned in Chapter 4, the best way to evaluate treatment outcomes is to compare notes and reports to baseline information. As we terminated therapy, I conducted an evaluation session with Ben and his parents. Before this session, I talked with the main figures in Ben's life. First, I talked with Ben's physical therapist. She mentioned that Ben did not talk with her, but reported that he looked happier, was no longer cynical or provocative, and that he had written to her once that he could talk, but not with her.

I returned to the kindergarten teacher. She said that during the school year, he did not talk with her, but she met him several times on his way back home from summer camp, and then he smiled and talked with her. Also, she said that before school started in the autumn, she took all the children to visit their new class. Ben talked just like all his peers.

The parents said that Ben was talking nonstop and that it was difficult to believe that he had ever had a problem.

In that evaluation session, Ben himself told me: "I can talk like everyone else. I'm okay."

Comparing Ben's behavior near the termination of treatment to the baseline data clearly demonstrated that Ben had overcome his problem of selective mutism. Also, although there were no baseline self-reports for comparison, Ben's records from the last few weeks of therapy indicated that he was inviting friends over, willing to go to visit friends, and taking part in social activities with his peer group. I could certainly affirm that his social behavior as well as his anxiety had improved and that he was functioning very well.

I continued meeting with Ben for a few more weeks, trying to empower him to be more confident, discussing his progress, and helping him understand that he was strong and capable.

Maintenance. At this point, in line with my routine practice in all cases of child therapy, I told Ben that, because of his significant improvement and change in behavior, his therapy was completed. We had achieved the goals of treatment. However, I explained that it was important for us to continue working together for a short while longer on learning how to reinforce and maintain these changes, so as to prevent regression and deal with the difficulties and challenges lying ahead. We were entering a new stage in our relationship; treatment was finished, and the maintenance and follow-up stage was beginning. In this new stage, we would continue meeting, but less often and partly by telephone.

I expected that renaming and redefining our therapeutic relationship would ease the separation process and enhance Ben's sense of empowerment and autonomy. In addition, I hoped that lasting contact during a follow-up period would foster Ben's commitment to continue charting his own behavior, in order to promote overlearning. In determining the frequency of contact, due to Ben's young age and limited time perception (see Table 4.9), I suggested that he call me once weekly at a predetermined time and report to me on his functioning. In our telephone conversations, I gradually instructed him to stop charting.

Two months later, Ben started school, and he acted like everyone else. At first, the mother had consulted me as to whether she should put him in a class where there would be no children he knew. I thought it was better not to interfere, and to let him enter the class where he was registered without informing the teacher about his past. There was no sign of a talking problem.

Ben invited me to the first school assembly of the first graders because he wanted me to hear him talking into the loudspeaker, reading a poem by a famous Israeli poet, Nathan Yonatan. If I may translate, the poem goes like this:

> When I look at the sky and my head is up,
> everyone thinks I am big and strong,
> but when I bend my head down no one sees me,
> and no one knows I exist....

7

Anxiety Disorder

LITERATURE REVIEW

Investigations of anxiety and fear in children have played a pivotal role in the development of theories of personality and psychopathology and in the development of interventions (Howard & Kendall, 1996). Fears and anxieties are the most prevalent mental illness in the United States (Thyer & Sowers-Hoag, 1988), and are widely recognized as the most common class of psychiatric disorders affecting children and adolescents (Albano et al., 1996; Donovan & Spence, 2000). A significant number of anxiety-disordered adults have reported suffering from symptoms of such disorders as children (Kendall, 1994).

Anxiety and fear should be evaluated in relation to the difference between normal behaviors and maladaptive ones, in view of their various definitions and criteria, in terms of their comorbidity with other childhood disorders, and in connection to age and gender criteria.

Normal Versus Maladaptive Behavior

As described in Part I, children are a population in a constant state of change. Hence, a behavior that appears normal could become problematic several months later, and, conversely, what seems to be problematic at present could change in the near future (Kazdin, 1988a; Ronen, 1993c, 1995). The transitory nature of most behavior problems supports spontaneous recovery as the rule in childhood. Studies of children who suffered from fears and anxiety but were not referred to therapy have often shown that such maladaptive behaviors emerge over the course of normal development (Lapouse & Monk, 1958; Werry & Quay, 1971). However, most fears disappear without consequence (Kazdin, 1988a). Seen from an ethnological perspective, fear and anxieties help children adapt to the world in which they live (Ronan & Deane, 1998). Anxiety in its adaptive form helps children begin to assimilate within a world of others. Moderate levels of anxiety can serve a regulatory function, helping children monitor behavior in accordance with social, academic, and cultural expectations (Ronan & Deane, 1998).

On the other hand, for a significant number of children, there is a probability that fears will be lifelong. As such, they might be handicapping or may impinge negatively on the routine developmental challenges of childhood. The anxiety experience may then become a stable negative force in their lives (Albano et al., 1996; Kendall et al., 1992).

Variance in Definitions

Anxiety is a broad concept that includes features of fear, phobia, and general or social anxieties. Careful evaluation of the child is imperative, especially due to recent changes in diagnostic categories (Manassis, 2000). Defining criteria is necessary to differentiate between normal fears and fears that are "too much" or maladaptive (Ronan & Deane, 1998). Fear is generally thought of as a discrete reaction to circumscribed stimuli, as a normal reaction, and as one usually outgrown. Anxiety is a more diffuse and internalized response. It is important to define the normal fears and anxieties that characterize normal behavior, in order to decide whether or not the specific behavior is deviant.

Comorbidity of Disorders

Different disorders frequently occur in the same child over time (Manassis, 2000). During the last decade, it has been suggested that a comorbidity of anxiety and depression exists in children and adolescents, and that both of these constitute variants of a single mood disorder (Brady & Kendall, 1992; Kazdin, 1994b).

Age Criteria

Fears and anxieties are found in children from infancy through adolescence, comprising a common part of normal growth. Those fears seen in infancy typically occur as a reaction to something occurring in the infant's environment, such as a loud voice, strangers, or bright light (Elbedour et al., 1997; Morris & Kratochwill, 1991; Silverman et al., 1995). As the child grows older, into the early school years, fears broaden and involve the dark, supernatural figures, and particular persons, objects, and events. Later on, fears turn to imaginary figures, objects, and events as well as to the future (Jersild, 1968). In middle childhood, one primary developmental task is socially based. Many of children's fears then are related to social events such as fears of new unfamiliar peers, going out to a party, or being accepted by friends. Many of the fears common in adolescence are related to their main age-related social tasks, developing their own self-identity and separating from the family.

Age criteria are usually relied upon to determine whether or not a particular behavior pattern is maladaptive, and it has been shown that many specific behavior problems are more prevalent among younger children (Kazdin, 1988a). While the trend for improvement with age is true for many disorders, it is even more emphasized when fears and anxieties are considered. Fear itself is an adaptive rather than maladaptive mechanism and may be necessary for normal children's development. Yet, as children mature, fears should diminish both in number and magnitude, thereby indicating adaptation to one's present environment.

Anxiety disorders in children and adolescents can be considered a silent epidemic. Their prevalence in the population has been reported to range between 6% and 18% (Velosa & Riddle, 2000). A number of studies have examined the incidence of children's fears within particular age ranges. However, much of the research is out of date or methodologically problematic. Jersild and Holmes (1935), for example, attempted to develop age norms for children's fears and found an average of 4.6 fears among children. Lapouse and Monk (1958) reported that, out of 482 children aged 7–12 years, 43% had seven or more fears. Ollendick (Ollendick, 1983; Ollendick et al., 1985) identified an even higher average of 13 fears among children and youth between the ages of 7 and 18. More recent studies have shown that internalized problems such as anxieties are found in 10–20% of school aged children (Anderson, 1994; Elbedour et al., 1997; Howard & Kendall, 1996).

Gender Criteria

Boys are known to outnumber girls in most behavior problems at a ratio of 2 : 1 (Kazdin, 1988a; Mash & Terdal, 1988). Yet, most studies on fears (e.g. Barrios & Hartman, 1988; Morris & Kratochwill, 1983) have observed higher anxiety levels among girls. Barrios and Hartman showed that girls usually tend to report a greater number of fears and anxieties than do boys. However, this trend might reflect girl's higher willingness to disclose negative feelings.

* * *

Fears are therefore age-related, transitory in nature, and of short duration. They vary in intensity both in any given child and from one child to another, and may be seen more prominently in girls than most other behavior problems (Elbedour et al., 1997).

Treatment

Early forms of therapy for childhood anxiety were borrowed from adult treatment models. More recently, the need has been recognized to design treatment from a child-based perspective (Barrett, 2000). Strauss (1988) noted a lack of empirical outcome evaluations for the treatment of anxiety disorders. Studies of childhood anxiety disorders have increased in recent years, but the clinical implications of the work are sometimes difficult to discern (Manassis, 2000).

Kendall (1994) presented his study as the first randomized clinical trial investigating the effectiveness of cognitive behavioral therapy for childhood anxiety disorders. Most of the existing behavioral techniques for children concern the treatment of specific childhood fears and phobias, and are based on case studies rather than on randomized control studies (Kanfer et al., 1975; King et al., 1988; Ronen, 1996a,b).

The most common treatments used for anxiety disorders today include family-based behavior therapy, parent training, individual-based cognitive behavioral therapy including relaxation and exposure therapy, or combined cognitive behavioral and drug therapy (Moore & Carr, 2000).

Increasing evidence supports cognitive behavioral treatment for anxiety disorders, alone or in combination with pharmacotherapy (Mannassis, 2000). Schroeder and Kendall (2000) reported the efficacy of both individual and group cognitive behavioral treatments in a controlled study comparing treatments to a waiting list.

The major methods of fear reduction in children's cognitive behavior therapy comprise systematic desensitization, contingency management procedures, modeling procedures, exposure techniques, and a range of cognitive techniques (Morris & Kratochwill, 1991).

Desensitization procedures. These involve exposing the child in small, graduated steps to the feared situation or event, while he or she is performing an activity that is antagonistic to anxiety (i.e. relaxation exercises). The treatment consists of teaching the child relaxation, developing an anxiety hierarchy, and confronting the anxiety with relaxation whether in imagination or *in vivo*. Few studies have related to the use of desensitization with children, and most of these were of single case design rather than controlled studies (Graziano, 1978; Graziano et al., 1979; King et al., 1988; Miller, 1979; Taylor, 1972).

Contingency management procedures. These are based on reinforcing the child while exposing him or her to the feared situation, in order to decrease the avoidance disorder and increase the frequency of performance (King et al., 1988; Leitenberg & Callahan, 1973; Morris & Kratochwill, 1991). In this technique, the child is given a specific, predetermined reinforcement each time he or she is ready to confront the fearful event. Most reinforcement techniques are combined with desensitization, exposure, or cognitive techniques.

Modeling procedures. Modeling treatments utilize the observation of a model who experiences positive behavior change and positive reinforcement while presenting the feared behavior. Studies have reported the efficacy of watching a positive model in order to reduce fears of dental treatment (White & Davis, 1974), test anxiety (Mann & Rosental, 1969), and snake avoidance (Ritter, 1968).

Exposure techniques. The most common treatment technique for anxiety disorders in adults consists of exposure therapy. Most of the other techniques described here also include elements of exposure during treatment. Exposure is based on: (a) rational explanations to clients concerning the need to expose themselves to threatening stimuli and to stop their avoidant behavior; (b) the pinpointing of exposure targets; (c) the rating of anxiety levels before, during, and immediately following exposure; (d) the ability to remain in the feared situation until the anxiety decreases; and (e) the request that throughout the entire procedure relatives or significant others avoid reassuring the client or reinforcing the avoidant response (Marks, 1969, 1978, 1987; Ronen, 1996b; Silverman et al., 1995).

With children, exposure treatment necessitates adaptation to their unique characteristics such as their irrational, concrete thinking and limited perceptions of time (Piaget, 1924). It is difficult for children to remain in a given situation for a long period even under pleasant circumstances, and far less so when the situation is aversive (Ronen, 1996b). Children might refuse to cooperate or to return for subsequent sessions, and exposure to very distressing situations could, under certain conditions, strengthen their fears (Redd et al., 1979). Ullmann and Krasner (1975) have warned therapists to implement exposure techniques very carefully with children in view of the possible negative experiences resulting from the anxiety-provoking scenes presented. Despite these liabilities, most of the existing knowledge on treating childhood anxiety disorders relates to exposure therapy as applied to specific fears or phobias (Ayllon et al., 1970; Kendall, 1994; Leitenberg & Callahan, 1973; Ronen, 1997b; Zikis, 1983).

In order to expose children, the therapist needs the full compliance not only of the child as a client, but also of the parents who usually reinforce the fears and anxieties. Children's fears often comprise reflections of their mothers' fears (Barrios & Hartman, 1988). Even when mothers are not anxious, it is very hard for them to avoid reinforcing their children's anxious reactions and to allow their children to expose themselves to feared situations, especially at the beginning of the treatment process, when crying or shouting may be the child's typical response. Thus, exposure treatment of children necessitates the design of a treatment program for the whole family.

Cognitive techniques. The range of cognitive techniques available for reduction of fears and anxiety includes self-instruction, relaxation, and self-exposure. Research on cognitive behavioral treatments for childhood anxieties has focused on nighttime fears, fear of dental/medical procedures, and test anxiety, presenting clinical case studies (Kendall, 1994). For example, Kanfer and colleagues (1975) used self-control procedures (self-talk) to treat children's nighttime fears. Ronen (1996b) designed an intervention package of self-control exposure therapy for children. Most of the studies of cognitive behavioral therapy with children reported treatment success in comparison to a control group, when using a coping skills approach that combined self-instructional techniques with behavioral techniques. The majority of existing cognitive behavioral programs involve elements of gradual exposure therapy combined with operant procedures, exposure in imagination (Thyer & Sowers-Hoag, 1988), social skills training, and self-control therapies (Ronen, 1996b).

Howard and Kendall (1996) reported the effectiveness of a family-based cognitive behavioral therapy in treating anxious children. They emphasized the importance of social negotiation processes in the treatment outcome. Focus was channeled on changes that were seen across the family, increased parental tolerance of children's negative affect, and reduced demands for perfect performance. Kendall and Chu (2000) described the efficacy of a treatment manual for anxiety disorders for children. They evaluated retrospective therapist ratings of the flexibility used when applying the procedures and strategies prescribed in the treatment manual (Kendall & Chu, 2000). They found that the manual could be very effective as long as the therapist could adopt the manual to the specific child's needs, developmental stage, and kind of fear reported.

The following case study utilized a full range of techniques to treat a child's fears, including exposure and modeling procedures, etc., but mostly cognitive–constructivist methods used creatively. Emphasis was placed on the creative integration of art, movement, metaphors, and experiential modes of therapy.

ARI'S FEAR OF WINTER, WINDS, AND THUNDERSTORMS

First Two Sessions: History and Assessment

When Ari entered my office for the first time, I almost could not see him. He came escorted by both his parents, who were tall, big people. His father, a security man, arrived armed. His mother, a physical education teacher, was almost as tall as her husband. Their son, aged 5 years and 10 months, was hidden between the two of them, barely reaching his parents' thighs. Ari was short and thin, and he talked so quietly that I had to sit down or bend over in order to hear him or to converse with him. When seated between his parents, Ari looked as if he had almost drowned and had difficulty making room for himself. Still, he declined to sit in another chair and preferred squeezing in between the two of them.

The parents told me that Ari was their firstborn child and that he had a 4-year-old sister who was already as tall as Ari. They said they came to me because Ari was "scared to death" whenever the wind would blow. He refused to leave home; he would not stay alone even in his own room; he kept standing by the windows watching the "poor miserable trees;" and he would frighten his younger sister about how they would both die soon, because the wind would destroy their house and carry them away. The winter had just started, and Ari's parents did not know how they would cope in the upcoming months.

In learning about his history, I discovered that Ari's family had lived abroad for the past five years and had returned to Israel only a few months earlier. The country where they had lived was famous for its powerful windstorms, and many times as Ari opened an umbrella, being as small and thin as he was, the wind would actually carry him away. Once, a storm had been so severe that he witnessed several trees crashing down, and since that time, he was afraid of "falling down like a tree."

During the entire first session with Ari and his parents, Ari's mother embraced him, looking as if she were shielding and protecting him, and often she answered instead of him when he had been asked a question. Whenever I asked Ari about his fears, his mother would reply, "Oh, we are afraid, aren't we?" and then she would nonverbally hint to me, pointing to her son's body as if she were saying, "What do you want? He's so tiny." It was clear that his mother was very worried about him being hurt. His father, on the other hand, wanted him to become stronger and had been pushing him to take a self-defense class like judo. Ari cried out, "But I hate all those activities!" During the session I discovered that, despite his age and normal intelligence, Ari was completely dependent on his parents to do everything for him, whether inviting friends over, talking with teachers whenever he had even the slightest problem, and picking out his clothes every morning. Ari seemed to be very shy, insecure, and lacking in self-confidence.

Due to Ari's young age, I determined that the assessment of his problem should be based mainly on the parents' verbal reports on his behavior (see Table 4.3). On the other hand, the emotional nature of his problem, with the goal of removing anxiety, required that information be gathered from Ari himself (see Table 4.2). In light of Ari's normal intelligence and high motivation for change (and his location on the cusp between early and middle childhood), direct assessment of Ari could also be added to the assessment battery, including direct observation of Ari's behavior in the clinic and projective tests such as drawing to assess his emotions. Therefore, at the end of the session, I asked Ari to come to the next meeting alone. His parents would of course bring him, but they would leave him with me and come to pick him up.

At this next session, Ari entered my office and found me sitting on the floor. I asked him to join me there, trying to meet him "on his own ground." I asked Ari about his friends, hobbies, and movies he used to watch on television. I was impressed with Ari as a thoughtful boy who had just started the first grade in school. I asked him to draw his family, and Ari drew two very large parental figures, a quite normally sized sister, and himself very small and vague. At the end of the session, I invited his parents to join us. I then asked Ari and his parents to chart his behavior over the next two weeks as baseline data, and I invited Ari to another session with me, after they had completed the baseline data collection.

Baseline assessment procedure. I asked the family to take records of Ari's behavior and the parents' responses concerning three main issues. Recording the first issue was mainly the parents' job. They were instructed to observe several behaviors as they currently were manifested in the family: who picked out Ari's clothes for school every day, whether they did things instead of him (such as talking with the teacher about extremely minor issues, calling to invite friends over), and any roles or chores that Ari took on in the family (such as throwing away the garbage, washing the dishes, etc). The second chart was assigned to Ari and his parents; they were asked to note any subject that Ari avoided, or any activity he refused to do or had to be forced to do. The third chart was Ari's alone, measuring his fears on a scale of 0–10. Ari determined that 0 (a "failing mark") meant his fears were extremely high, while 10 (a "perfect score") meant he was not at all afraid.

Analyzing the baseline data. After two weeks of baseline recording, Ari and his parents came to the clinic and presented their charts. The first chart showed that over the baseline period Ari never initiated taking on responsibility for himself or his family, and his parents never asked him to. During these two weeks, they took Ari to school each day, but Ari would not even enter his classroom alone, and the parents had to escort him until he sat down at his own desk. Twice they went into the school to talk with his teacher, because Ari would not dare talk to her, once to explain why Ari was late to school one morning, and the second time to explain why he did not bring a pencil to class when asked. Five times the mother called and invited friends over to visit with Ari, and he never called a friend on his own. Each morning she was the one to prepare his clothes for school, and each night she prepared his pajamas for him while he went to take a shower. Not once did the parents ask him to do chores such as clearing off the dinner table, taking out the trash, or tidying his room. It was clear that they never allowed or encouraged Ari to be independent or try coping alone, and they often talked about him as weak, needing help, and being unable to do things.

The second chart, filled out by Ari and his parents together, revealed that during these two weeks, Ari was restless, especially at night, and refused to sleep alone in his bed, in case a storm would commence. It should be noted that during this two-week period coinciding with the early winter season, there were many occasions of rain and wind gusts, and several electrical outages for a few minutes each. In the afternoons, Ari never let his mother out of sight. He cried a great deal when she went into another room and did not let him come with her. Yet, he was also afraid of accompanying her out of the house, and he refused to go out to visit friends in their homes. Taking him to school was a difficult task each morning, involving crying and yelling.

In the third chart, Ari rated his fears each day as being at the top of the scale, between 9 and 10.

Next, as described in Chapter 4, I undertook the phases of decision making that encompass assessment of the intake information, evaluation of the problem, design of the intervention process, and evaluation and maintenance of treatment outcomes.

Phase 1 of Decision Making: Does Ari Need Therapy or Not?

Following the guidelines for making treatment decisions presented in Chapter 4, I first assessed whether or not Ari's problem necessitated intervention. Relating to the problem variables, fears in general are very common among children. However, it can be seen that Ari's problem was not a regular, normal, developmental fear. Rather, it appeared to be a fear that had become broader and more extensive and had caused him to develop avoidance behavior. In addition, the fear had shown no improvement since its onset; to the contrary, it had only worsened. Ari's specific storm-related anxieties had generalized to many other areas. Moreover, the parents' inability to allow him to cope alone with everyday tasks and challenges had contributed to the maintenance of Ari's general helplessness and dependence. Therefore, it appeared that Ari was at risk for developing even more severe avoidance disorders and further generalization.

An examination of developmental variables showed that this fear was deviant among children in Ari's age or sex group and was not common in his environment. A look at the child and family variables revealed that both Ari and his parents were suffering as a result of Ari's disorder. His fears disturbed their normal functioning and limited some of the family's activities. The parents were worried about his future and wished to resolve the problem. Ari himself was suffering and seemed motivated to work toward change.

The treatment characteristics pinpointed the good prognosis that exists for fears, anxieties, and phobias when treated and the known effectiveness of treatments in this area. At the same time, it could be predicted that Ari's problem would not disappear without treatment, and that its elimination would significantly change the child's future.

Altogether, these considerations clearly indicated the need to treat Ari's fears.

Phase 2 of Decision Making: Classifying Ari's Referral and Goals for Change

Phase 2 of decision making (see Chapter 4) concerns the classification of children's referred disorders in terms of the goals of intervention and developmental considerations. As related to the four main types of referral, Ari's disorder could be classified as the third type: the need to remove anxiety (see Table 4.2). This kind of classification pinpoints overcontrolled children, who are afraid of losing control, are overanxious, and suffer from fears and phobias that cause them to avoid social situations and become withdrawn in their behavior. Relating to this classification, Ari's disorder necessitated the acquisition of coping skills, and it was determined that the treatment should be conducted to target change in his behavior as well as in his emotions and thoughts.

Relating to developmental considerations, Ari was at the stage of early childhood (see Table 4.3). At this stage, his main social tasks were to start coping with academic as well as social roles. Anxiety and fears at this stage were liable to prevent the child from becoming involved in social and academic assignments that were important for his healthy growth. Fears could prevent Ari from participating in peer group activities, visiting friends, or even just leaving the house to play. These features clearly emphasized the need to help Ari overcome his fears and be able to live like other children his age.

Phase 3 of Decision Making: Selecting Who Should Be Treated

This phase of decision making identifies who should be targeted for treatment, based both on Ari's problem area and developmental stage (Tables 4.5 and 4.4, respectively). Ari was almost 6 years old at the time of referral, the stage of early childhood when thinking is just emerging from the pre-operational level and is still concrete. He was dependent on his parents and needed to acquire early academic and social skills for independent functioning. Therapy for Ari's age group and for children with anxious behavior is usually applied to the family or to the child in the parents' presence, with an emphasis on supervising and counseling the parents. In Ari's case, I came to some conclusions based on the first two sessions, relating to Ari's physique and his fears, that facilitated my decision regarding how the treatment setting should be designed and who should be the targeted client.

With respect to Ari's body: First, it was true that Ari was a very slender, tiny boy, and his appearance increased his insecurity, but that was something Ari should learn to live with and accept. Second, his weakness also reflected his mother's concern and would not be resolved as long as the mother's fears were not treated. Third, Ari's father placed central emphasis in his life and career on physical strength, and pushed Ari to develop his own body shape. Ari, having a different personality, had been anxious and afraid of not satisfying his father's wishes.

Ari's fears could be understood in two ways. One was his lack of exposure to new experiences. His mother, by shielding him, escorting him, and protecting him, reinforced his fear of the unknown. He found it hard even to stand still and look at storm-caused damage, which was something he had been strenuously protected against. Ari had a model of parents who needed to be in full control of their lives. Ari felt unable to fully control what was going around him (i.e. the wind that blew against his will prevented him from being in control of his actions 100% of the time and made him aware of the fact that he could be carried away). This feeling frightened him as well as his parents. He and his parents needed help accepting the fact that not everything in life can and should be controlled.

The other way of understanding Ari's fears was to examine his way of thinking and the belief system that led him to develop misconceptions. From birth, being brought up as the first son of such big, athletic parents, he developed core ideas such as: "In this world one must be strong and big" and "Life is one big war, and you have to be strong enough to fight it." As he started developing his own self-image and self-esteem, Ari's automatic negative thoughts were: "I am small, I won't survive" and "I can't be what my parents are, I will fail." Ari felt inferior, incompetent, and worthless.

Whenever a child's treatment is concerned, the parents are involved, and very rarely can children accept, overcome, and cope with behaviors that go against their parents' will. However, my assessment of Ari's parents and their interaction with their son suggested that parental supervision would be of prime importance in this case. I therefore determined that the first step of intervention should involve counseling the parents separately, as a couple (not in a parents' group), in order to help them to:

1. Accept Ari as he was, as different from them, and let him grow up and develop to become what he would and not what they thought he should be.
2. Decrease their worries and enable them to "free" Ari by helping them see him take on responsibilities and cope with new experiences without being stopped by them.
3. Understand the side effects Ari experienced as a result of their concerns, which maintained the problem.

At the same time, the extent of Ari's storm related fears, the severity of his separation anxiety, and the persistent effect of his anxieties on his independent functioning indicated that parental counseling alone would be insufficient to resolve these problems. It was clearly apparent that Ari's fears would not disappear without direct exposure, indicating the need for Ari himself to also receive individual treatment.

My impression led me to use a multiple intervention within a single case design. A multiple intervention means that, following a general baseline assessment, two or more interventions are implemented subsequent to one another, such that they are not in effect at the same time (Kazdin, 1982). While applying one intervention related to one problem, the others are held in wait. The main reason for applying a multiple intervention is when assessment points to multiple needs for one client. A multiple intervention design can aim at changing one main behavior of a single client via several techniques or can aim at changing several main behaviors via several techniques. The major purpose of the design is to show that the client performs differently under different treatment conditions and that a change can be observed only in one specific behavior while implementing a specific intervention (Kazdin, 1982, 1994a).

Treatment efficacy in a multiple intervention design is evaluated for all of the applied interventions, in their sequence; it is not possible to evaluate the interventions separately. The efficacy of the intervention is proven when a gradual change in a targeted behavior is shown relative to the implementation of a specific intervention, while nontargeted behaviors remain stable (e.g. only Ari's independence is changed while supervising his parents, but his fears continue unchanged). The whole change that is desired comprises a combination of all the different interventions.

I decided to conduct a multiple intervention design for Ari, including three main settings (with Ari's and his parents' agreement), each addressing a different problem: parental counseling, individual child therapy, and working with the whole family. Parent counseling would focus on helping Ari's parents "let go," by giving him responsibilities, allowing him to be independent, and refraining from doing things for him. Later on, the second intervention would concentrate on individual therapy with Ari, helping him become exposed to his fears, stop his avoidance behavior, improve his coping, and develop self-confidence. The third intervention would be family therapy, aimed at helping the family to accept Ari as he was, and at fostering his self-confidence and sense of security within the family environment.

Phase 4 of Decision Making: Selecting Ari's Optimal Treatment Modes

According to my proposed guidelines, the next and final step in decision making prior to intervention concerns determining how the therapy should be conducted. In deciding which modes and techniques should be selected for Ari, a number of therapist, child, developmental, and problem variables required consideration. Regarding the goals of treatment, Ari's problem was an internalizing, emotional one, relating to the third type of referral – removal of anxiety. Treating Ari's parents would be based on verbal counseling to address their thoughts, emotions, and behaviors in an effort to help them improve their style of childrearing with Ari. However, because the problem consisted of anxiety, individual treatment of Ari would use various techniques to address several goals. Exposure exercises (actual practicing) would aim to help him stop his avoidance behavior, and he would have to face the things he feared. Indirect methods such as drawing, movement, imagery, and stories would help him change his thoughts and emotions. Due to Ari's concrete thinking and the need for practical exercises at his age, the exposure treatment was designed to involve indirect modes such as drawing, movement therapy, and play therapy, rather than being based only on the exposure assignment itself (like in adult therapy).

First Stage of Multiple Treatment: Counseling Ari's Parents

After the intake sessions, I started meeting with Ari's parents. My aim was to help them accept Ari as he was, by facilitating their ability to clarify their expectations, identify the differences between them and their son, and unearth his positive strengths, skills, and abilities.

In the first session, we focused on their belief system relating to Ari and their expectations from him. I asked them to draw a picture of Ari as he was. Then, they were asked to draw him as they wished him to be in ten years. After a few first minutes of hesitation, they did so. I selected this nonverbal technique mainly because they were both trying to deny the way they overprotected Ari and were using verbalizations to justify that. I thought that a nonverbal technique would detour around their rationalizations and enable them to face their real emotions concerning Ari.

In drawing Ari as he was, each parent sketched an outline of Ari as a very small figure in the corner of the page. The father drew Ari without facial expression, and the mother sketched a neutral one. In drawing him as they wished him to be in ten years, the father placed the page vertically and filled it with a sketch of his son kicking a soccer ball. When asked to describe his drawing, the father depicted a tall, strong, athletic, popular boy. The mother's detailed drawing of her future son was on one-third of a horizontal page, portraying a normally sized figure smiling and holding balloons on strings; she said she wanted a happy, independent boy who was satisfied with himself.

This task was important in clarifying my own as well as their understanding of how they perceived Ari currently versus what they wished him to be; to determine what they felt was missing in order for the present Ari to become what they desired; and to evaluate if these perceptions and wishes were truly helpful to them or their son. As a homework assignment, both of them were asked to write down Ari's current strengths and good points.

During the second session, based on self-monitoring and self-evaluation that emerged from a review of their homework assignment, we focused on the way they valued their son's wisdom as well as his charm and even his manipulative ability, which they viewed as advantageous. The couple was instructed in how to help Ari by encouraging him to do things independently such as talk with his teacher directly about minor issues when necessary, call a friend, or help around the house. The third and fourth sessions in parent counseling focused on the impact of their role, reinforcing the parents' motivation and ability to let Ari cope on his own and instructing them in how to continue working with him to maintain the outcomes achieved.

Immediately after the first month of parent counseling, even before starting therapy with Ari, some improvements were shown in Ari's functioning. While his fears did not lessen, he did begin acting more independently. For example, he started picking out his own clothes before school; he took the initiative to call his friends when he wanted them to come over; he was the one to close the windows when it started raining and he was scared; and he stopped saying "I can't do that because I'm too small" all the time. He was even willing to enter his classroom alone (after being brought to school by his mother). According to the mother, his teacher also mentioned that, for the first time, Ari was talking with her and had even asked her a question. Prior to that time, the teacher's sole conversations were with Ari's mother, not with him.

After this first month, I started seeing Ari every week individually, and I continued supervising his parents in sessions every 2–3 weeks. The sessions with the parents focused on analyzing Ari's progress, trying to evaluate the reasons for that progress, and reinforcing the parents' ability to allow him to grow up and become independent.

Second Stage of Multiple Treatment: Individually Treating Ari

As mentioned above, working with Ari's parents did improve his independent functioning but did not change his fears, in line with the principles underlying the multiple intervention design. Now, individual treatment began, focusing on Ari's fears and anxieties. Based on Phase 4 of the decision making process, the fact that Ari was in early childhood and needed to remove anxieties pinpointed the importance of treating Ari using a combination of nonverbal, verbal, and experiential methods that entailed many demonstrations, examples, and play assignments. I incorporated these methods into my self-control intervention model (SCIM), as detailed in Chapter 5.

SCIM module 1: Cognitive restructuring and redefinition. My first aim while treating Ari was to help him change his emotions and thoughts. Young children find it hard to differentiate thoughts from emotions. When asked what they think, they may answer, "I'm afraid," and when asked what they feel, they may say, "That this is very bad."

Ari's thoughts and belief systems, purporting that wind and movement were bad and dangerous, were well rooted in his past. Changing these misconceptions through verbal therapy would not be very effective because of his ability to use arguments and persuasive tactics as to why his way of thinking was right. I believed that only by changing Ari's way of feeling would he be able to change his way of thinking. Then he could construct a new meaning for his life, to change the way he looked at himself, and to become able to expose himself to feared situations. This change in thoughts, beliefs, and self-efficacy was the objective of the exposure sessions.

Our first individual session was a planned walk outside the clinic. Ari's fears were based on his automatic thoughts: that trees were miserable; that they were constantly being punished by the wind, and that they were afraid of winter. His fears made him avoid exposure to the anxiety-provoking situation. Taking Ari outside had two main purposes. First, as Mahoney (1991) proposed, in order to better understand what it is like to be the person we serve, we need to experience the self, the world, and the emotions that characterize the client's life. Second,

I expected that exposure and experiential methods could help change his misconceptions more than verbal intervention would. I wanted Ari to feel and sense the environment; I wanted him to look around and try to find out whether it was the trees that were afraid or whether it was his own fears that he saw reflected in the trees.

On our walk (which took place on a winter day in the clinic's neighborhood), we observed the trees, trying to note if they looked happy or sad, had enough water or were dry, whether or not they had leaves, and what they did when the wind blew. Ari looked around and touched the trees. At my request, he spoke as if he were the trees' voices, expressing what he expected the trees might say. His homework assignment for that week was to look at trees in his home and school environments, trying to understand the trees' feelings and differentiating these from his own feelings (e.g. he might say, "Hey, the tree looks happy! Its leaves are all green and there are new leaves growing. Why am I afraid? That tree isn't afraid").

In light of Ari's sensitivity and the fact that his language was peppered with images, metaphors, and expressions that sounded like he was "talking in pictures," I thought it would be best to utilize this language in treatment. People's conceptual systems play a central role in defining their everyday realities (Kopp, 1995). I decided to concentrate on metaphor techniques beginning in the first session. Human beings are largely metaphorical in the way they think, what they do, and what they experience every day (Lakoff & Johnson, 1980). Metaphors are helpful in therapy by reframing people's viewpoints, transporting us into the less tangible domains of life as a journey and as a story to be told (Carlsen, 1995). Metaphors facilitate the remaking of our life stories.

I shared with Ari a metaphor I use while working with elderly people, emphasizing the different shapes and qualities of the trees in every season, so that each season has its own beauty to be enjoyed. In spring, leaves are budding and new life starts, and one feels the happiness exuding from the color and the new beginning. Then, as summer comes, the leaves continue to mature, providing a rich green canopy to protect us from the sun. When autumn arrives, the trees display a whole array of colors that are often breathtaking. Winter trees are often seen as a sign of barrenness and death, but winter also provides the opportunity to see the structure of the tree, the way it really is. Its shape, its branches, and its surrounding can be truly appreciated. Then, the snow brings out another beauty, covering the trees with a white blanket. Winter gives opportunity for the new life, which begins anew in the spring.

After describing the metaphor, I asked Ari to draw the trees in different seasons and to discuss which of them he liked the most.

In the next session (still aiming at changing misconceptions), we watched a part of the video film of Walt Disney's *Mary Poppins* (Walsh, 1997). During our viewing, I tried to help Ari pinpoint his feelings when it was raining or when the gusts of wind blew. I wanted Ari to notice what Mary Poppins felt during the wind and how fun it was for her to be carried away by the wind.

After working on cognitive restructuring, it was clear that although Ari still suffered from fears, he had begun to think differently. He started to accept the fact that maybe wind was not that terrible, that there might even be some fun to winter and rain, and that maybe in the future he could learn to control his fears. I encouraged him to use self-talk ("I know I can do it," "Hey, this is actually fun," or "I really can handle this") in encountering inclement weather and new situations.

SCIM module 2: Problem analysis. In the second module of the self-control model, I wanted Ari to see how his way of thinking about the wind had affected the way he felt and had culminated in his avoidance behavior. I wanted him to try and see that, by changing the way he thought about winter, he could change and control his fears.

I told Ari about the connection between his brain and his body, introducing illustrations of the human body and indicating how the brain sends commands to the body. I explained how his thoughts (e.g. "the trees are miserable") elicited his fears (e.g. "it's terrible, so I'm scared"), which were linked to his behaviors (e.g. crying and restlessness). We exercised different kinds of analysis to show him the strength of his thoughts and the links between thoughts, emotions, and behaviors. For example, we tried to see what would happen if Ari could tell himself: "Winter is wonderful for the trees," or "The rain is necessary for the flowers to grow," or "I am stronger than the trees," and then try to guess which emotions and behaviors would follow those new thoughts. He was also asked to keep a record of his attempts to change automatic negative thoughts (e.g. "How terrible, it's raining") into mediated positive ones (e.g. "What fun it is to dance in the rain").

SCIM module 3: Attentional focus. In the next module, I wanted to teach Ari to listen to his internal cues and to identify specific details of his feelings about the wind, such as the kinds of physical sensations he experienced while afraid and their location in his body. Ari was asked to record at home what he felt when the wind blew, when it rained, or when there was lightning. He was asked to write down in which part of his body he felt it, what exactly he felt, and how strong it was. When Ari came back to the next session, he showed me his charts. He noted that he had located his fears as mainly in his stomach (he felt stomachaches) and in his throat and eyes (which hurt when he started crying). I had also asked him to record at home the intensity of his fears, on the same 0–10 scale used during the baseline assessment. He showed me that he had rated himself at the top of the scale (10) almost every day, indicating intense fear. In addition, I brought an actual ladder into the clinic that day, for Ari to use as a scale to measure his fear level during our sessions. Ari determined that the floor represented a safe haven, and the top of the ladder represented the most terrifying of his fears. As he progressed up the rungs of the ladder during treatment, he felt more and more in control of his terror.

We also focused on increasing Ari's sensitivity to his internal stimuli utilizing movement therapy methods. In the earlier sessions, Ari had learned to identify his thoughts and feelings, and to realize that others could feel differently than he. Now, we tried to play "as if." Believing that Ari's problem was caused and maintained by his strong emotions, I planned for him to "live" the feared situation once again, becoming aware of the emotions it elicited. However, this time, I wanted him to be able to ask himself if the feelings he felt really reflected the emotions natural to the situation or if they could be different. To this end, Ari needed to expose himself over and over to the exploration and experiencing of wind, winter, and rain.

In the safe environment of my clinic, I placed a large fan to make the air move, and, in a modeling exercise, both Ari and I played the role of trees moving in a storm and trying to feel what it was like to be pushed about. At first, Ari acted as if he were at war. He started fighting against the wind, trying to stop his hair from blowing around, trying to stick to his ground and not move his feet. Then, frustrated from the fight, he fell down, starting to cry and complain about how much his body hurt him. Looking up at me enjoying the wind, his expression suddenly changed, and he started laughing. Getting up as a tree and moving his arms slowly as branches, Ari said, "Oh, wonderful. All summer long I had to stay still. It's so good to move." Ari was the first one to say, "Oh, this is fun."

Attentional focus and increasing sensitivity to internal cues help clients become more aware of themselves as well as to learn and accept themselves, and thus to increase their ability for change, self-confidence, and coping. Next, in trying to help Ari accept himself through movement methods, I asked him to try concentrating on his feelings and to make his movements bigger and bigger, learning to enjoy the movement and the change, instead of trying to keep still and reject it. We kept alternating roles, from being the wind to being a tree. Toward the end of the session, Ari asked to be "a small boy walking in the wind." That was the first time he did not fight against the wind but rather went with it, jumping, falling, rolling over, and enjoying the scene. Ari even started talking about how good the wind was for the small trees that could move from side to side, and how sorry he felt for the big trees that were too old to move and enjoy it. During this session, he also found an Indian rain stick in my room and, when he heard what it was, asked to borrow it. At home that week, Ari started dancing a rain dance and watching for rain, and even taught his sister to do the same.

Part of increasing Ari's attention was to notice changes in his own emotions as well as in the environment. Ari was instructed to walk around his neighborhood, find leaves that had fallen to the ground, put them in a booklet, and take note of their different colors and shapes. To further enhance Ari's internal focus and assist him in coping with states of anxiety, I suggested to him simple relaxation exercises such as trying to make his arm heavy or light, to lie down and relax his body, etc.

Up to now, we had concentrated on the first three modules: cognitive restructuring, rational analysis of the links between his problem, brain, and body, and attentional focus. After learning to change his way of thinking, to link behaviors to emotions and thoughts, and to increase awareness of his internal sensations, Ari was ready to begin working on the fourth skill module, exercising self-control.

SCIM module 4: Self-control exercises. The next two sessions targeted empowerment. Empowerment was achieved via training Ari to exercise self-control techniques in order to accept himself as a small person. Ari was directed to try to make the most out of himself, his fate, and his reality. He was asked to check if he really felt inferior, or if he only thought he should be inferior because of others' expectations from him. Gradually, Ari had already started developing self-confidence. Because Ari knew how to read and write, I assigned him the homework task of examining some books, finding some great people in our history who were physically small, and reading about them. Ari asked his parents to help him with their encyclopedia and to take him to the library. They read about Napoleon and Ben Gurion, and Ari came to the next session describing how some of the greatest people were "not tall at all, they even looked very small." Ari also started recognizing some benefits of his height using self-talk and self-instruction (e.g. "I can easily run away from Dad," "I'm very flexible," and "I will hide from the teacher"). At the same time, he became able to express expectations from himself that were unrelated to his size (e.g. "to be smart, maybe become an architect because I like to change things"). At this stage of treatment, Ari was asked to expose himself to real wind and rain outdoors. Not only did Ari overcome his fear of inclement weather, but his mother complained that he kept opening the windows throughout storms, watching the trees, and talking to them.

As we progressed with the different steps of the modules, it was clear that Ari was improving his coping and reducing his fears. His ratings of his fears decreased on his charts, and, during the sessions, he was able to climb up to the top rung of the ladder. His crying decreased, and his readiness to go outside, look at the rain, and leave the windows open changed remarkably.

Third Stage of Multiple Treatment: Working with the Family Unit

Ari had progressed in two major areas, increasing his independence following the parents' counseling and reducing his fears following individual treatment. I next focused through family therapy on the problem areas that had not shown a change. Ari was still very shy, his self-confidence was low, and he felt insecure within his family.

I therefore invited the whole family to four sessions, including Ari, his sister, and their parents. Those last sessions focused on how different each family member was from the others and how this diversity could contribute to mutual enjoyment gained from the different roles and places everyone had in the family. Knowing that the referred problem had been decreased, I felt it was important to work toward increasing positive coping and adaptive behaviors. Exercising self-evaluation and self-reinforcement methods, I wanted to encourage each member of the family to take responsibility for his or her own behavior, and to learn to let the others cope in their own ways. I believed that by finding his place in the family, Ari would feel better and improve his self-acceptance and self-esteem.

To demonstrate these concepts, I asked everyone in the family to talk and behave like someone else in the family. They all cooperated, imitating each other, laughing and exaggerating, and exchanging seats. Ari and his sister started making fun of their parents. Ari chose to talk like his mother, overemphasizing the way she always worried about him: "Ari, don't walk in the street. Someone might look at you. Ari, don't laugh! You might get a stomachache." The mother then asked, laughing, if she was that terrible and discussed it with the children. Both Ari and his sister tried to reach an agreement with their mother. They asked the mother to give them more freedom and try not to be as anxious as she usually was, while their father supported them very happily by commenting that "it's about time for her to let them grow up." In another exercise, I asked each of them, "Who would you like to be instead of yourself?" No one wanted to exchange places with another.

As a reinforcement exercise, I asked Ari's sister to compliment him. She said, "It was so fun to dance the rain dance with you. You're a great dancer. Will you dance with me again?" The fact that her compliment centered on Ari's physical ability attested to the change in Ari's body image as well as in the family atmosphere that had toned down expectations for Ari to grow into a strong athlete. We continued by having everyone compliment the others in the family and focus on their good characteristics. They were asked to continue this exercise at home by complimenting each other every day on one good thing they had done that day.

Another exercise was the "supermarket game of characteristics." All the family members had to try and sell some of their own attributes that they did not like much; for example, the mother tried to sell some of her anxiety. At the same time, the players had to try to purchase qualities they were lacking. It emerged that the father wanted to buy some sensitivity from Ari, the sister wanted to buy his sense of humor, and the mother wanted to buy his courage.

By the end of these sessions, it seemed as if each of the four family members was better able to talk to, accept, and express affection with the others, and the parents reported that Ari was feeling much more secure and confident.

Phase 5 of Decision Making: Evaluating Ari's Progress at the End of Therapy and Maintaining Treatment Outcomes

Evaluation. As seen in Chapter 4, evaluation of treatment outcomes is usually conducted by comparing baseline notes and reports to those at the end of therapy. The sources I used for Ari's evaluation included the teacher's report, the parents' report, and Ari's report, as well as my own impressions from the changes that had occurred in his behavior.

The teacher reported that a big change could be noted in Ari's behavior. He was not as shy as he used to be, he was involved with the other children during school recesses, he was talking with her, and he was even daring to ask her for things he needed.

As for the family reports, when I asked the parents to evaluate their son's progress, they started laughing. Ari's father said that now Ari did not ever seem to want to stay at home; he wanted to go to friends' houses every afternoon, and this had caused some problems because of the cold, wintry weather. Sometimes the parents did not want him to go out in heavy rainstorms for fear that he would catch a cold. When I showed them their baseline charts, Ari and his parents were surprised to see how much Ari had improved over the weeks of Ari's intervention. We reviewed each component of the baseline reports and very easily noted the changes in each as compared to Ari's charts at the end of therapy.

In the last family session, Ari's happiness, comfort level, and sense of confidence were clearly evident in every aspect of his being, in his verbal and nonverbal behavior, indicating that formal evaluation questionnaires were unnecessary.

This was a short-term therapeutic intervention designed to impart self-control skills to Ari and his family. After changing his thoughts and increasing his awareness, self-control exercises with Ari targeted overcoming fears, teaching him self-talk, using self-monitoring to record the change, and self-evaluation. Ari's parents learned to accept their child as-is, let him behave independently, and trust him. I am not sure if this process sufficed in order to modify Ari's feelings of inferiority forever, but I do know that he left therapy feeling much better with himself. He was no longer afraid of the wind; his parents stopped forcing him to become someone he was not; and he had found a voice for himself as a different but valuable person.

Using the multitreatment baseline single case design enabled me to analyze not only the changes in Ari, but also which intervention was responsible for each change. It was clear that, as we started working in parental counseling, Ari's independent functioning improved. The parents' report showed Ari's increased initiative to go out to friends' and to deal with his own fearful behavior (e.g. by closing the windows instead of waiting for his parents to do it for him, and by being ready to leave home without crying). However, his fear of the winter was not reduced until I started working individually with Ari and focusing on the self-control model for removing anxiety. Then, although the fear reduction did improve his coping, it was evident that these changes had not affected his low self-confidence. The family was very caring and supportive. Therefore, while receiving my supervision they were ready to comply with the instruction and let Ari take responsibility and cope. Working with the family helped in changing their attitude toward

Ari. The change in the family behavior facilitated Ari's ability to improve his self-esteem and stop viewing himself as weak and incompetent.

This case study highlights several important points. First, it emphasizes the fact that although they may seem to be simple problems, children's disorders comprise a combination of several components, and very rarely are they developed or maintained by one cause. Therefore, one solid intervention often does not help resolve the problem as well as an integrated intervention. As mentioned before, children's treatment usually involves several settings. This case demonstrates how each setting uniquely caused a change in one main behavior, and only the combination of all the settings (parent counseling, individual therapy, and family therapy) yielded the desired full change in all aspects of need. Furthermore, the fact that while focusing on one setting, only one specific behavior changed but not the others points to the fact that, while these behaviors are interrelated, each of them must be addressed directly in order to achieve effective change. The intervention as a whole showed that self-control training is effective for children and families in changing fearful behavior, overdependence, and low self-acceptance

Maintenance. I asked Ari to call me once a week over the next month in the follow-up period, in order to enhance generalization of his new self-control skills (see Table 4.9). I suggested to Ari that he take what he had already learned in treatment and try to apply it independently to other areas such as social problems (his shyness to invite a friend over) and problems with his parents. Over the next two years, either Ari or his mother would call me once every several months to update me on Ari's social and academic functioning. It was always a pleasure to hear how well he was coping and adjusting.

Just before ending this book, I coincidentally met Ari and his mother at his elementary school, when I went to see another client of mine. It was already two years after the end of our treatment. They told me that not only was Ari not afraid any more, but he was the one to initiate and organize the activities of his peers on Friday nights. He had also just returned from a mathematics competition for students in the region, and he had won first place. He had no problem participating in the contest and was able to stand up in front of all the other schools and answer the questions. Ari told me he had "long forgotten that stupidity of being afraid."

8

Traumatized Children

LITERATURE REVIEW

Throughout their development, children are exposed to a wide variety of events such as change, crisis, stress, and trauma. Those events may be personal (accidents, illness), familial (loss of relatives, economic difficulties, divorce), or environmental in nature. The latter include natural disasters (floods, earthquakes) or manmade adversities (war, murder, abuse). The diversity of such events significantly complicates the study of children's responses.

The concept of trauma has become the ultimate umbrella concept that organizes all the events that children experience and integrates danger, risk, crisis, stress, and harmful situations under one generalized definition. The ever-widening use of the concept of trauma, like that of many other technical terms, has led to a blurring of meaning and loss of conceptual precision (Brandell, 1992).

Psychoanalytic theory has distinguished three different conditions of trauma: traumatic neurosis, traumatic anxiety, and the posttraumatic neurotic-like state (Brandell, 1992). Other therapies, such as behavior, cognitive, or constructivist, view trauma as the child's response to external stimuli that harms him or her (Ronen, 1996b; Swell, 1995).

Traumatic experiences among children have always been a major concern of therapists. Traditionally, such experiences have been divided into two kinds: (a) natural disasters and dangers, such as hurricanes, floods, or earthquakes; sickness, death and (b) manmade disasters and dangers such as war, automobile accidents, and criminal acts such as burglaries and murders. In both these kinds of traumatic events, the child is usually seen as a victim of the environment or the society but one who can obtain the protection of his or her own family.

Recently, especially over the last two decades, a third kind of traumatic experience has gained much attention from therapists, educators, and legislators: child abuse. Child abuse comprises a manmade trauma that jeopardizes the child's future and causes injury in the present. Children of all ages, even infants, can be victims of abuse, in general, and sexual abuse, in particular. Reported rates for child abuse range from 10% to 23% of the child population (Knell, 1993). In general, boys are abused less frequently than girls (particularly with regard to sexual abuse). However, there is reason to believe that the incidence for boys may be higher than reported (Knell, 1993). Out of the abused children reported, 54% had experienced the abuse at home by a family member (Bowen, 2000).

Children's responses to traumatic events vary as a function of the kind of event they experienced, as well as the child's personal characteristics and available support systems. Sometimes children who experience traumatic events (whether social, environmental, familial, or personal) develop an inability to continue life normally and begin to elicit a broad range of symptoms and disorders. For example, a child whose parents are killed in a car accident may develop immediate, long lasting sleep disturbances, diurnal and nocturnal enuresis, and difficulties in academic adjustment. Such symptoms may pose a risk to children's well being and jeopardize their future growth and development (Garbarino et al., 1991). In other words, such responses might lead to socially or personally handicapping emotional disorders (Garmezy & Rutter, 1985) and permanent psychological scars (Pynoos & Nader, 1988). The issue of how trauma, crisis, and stressful experiences affect children's development has raised contradictory findings. The studies have focused on several questions. One question focuses on whether it is the child's internal responses or the situational cues that influence his or her behavior (Rahav & Ronen, 1994). Another one is that whether children develop post trauma disorders, or do they view the trauma as a challenge they have to cope with, and develop new skills. Wiszinckas (1982) suggested that a situational crisis is a dangerous opportunity to which a child may either succumb through symptom development, or emerge with increased strength and mastery.

Children's Response to Trauma

Insufficient studies and knowledge are available concerning children's behavior following trauma (Peuler, 1988). Therefore, the understanding of children's responses to such events must depend on the varying studies of trauma existing in the literature. Traumagenic factors are said to be common to all victims of traumatic experiences and abuse, but will manifest themselves differently in each child. Frequent symptoms of young children cited in the literature include nightmares and sleep disturbances, regression in toileting and other skills, expressions of anger and fear, eating disorders, and sexualized behaviors (Kendall-Tackett et al. 1993). A high incidence has been documented of attention deficit hyperactive disorder (ADHD) and oppositional defiant behavior, as well as other kinds of adjustment disorders, among children with a history of abuse (Ford et al., 2000).

Epidemiological studies have revealed the high frequencies of disorders among children who experienced traumatic episodes. The frequency of problem behaviors reported by children during stressful episodes was found to be significantly related to their pre-stress frequency of problem behaviors (Anderson et al., 1987; Rahav & Ronen, 1994). Most studies reported more behavior problems among those who had shown more pre-stress problems.

The Environmental Approach

The first research trend, depicting an environmental approach, proposes that the kind of environmental change and stress experienced is the most important component influencing children's disorders. War, disaster, hurricane, or flooding all influence children's behavior differently than would being abused by their family members. This trend accentuates the environment's mediating role in the development of children's responses. Throughout childhood, children are constantly exposed to different kinds of changes: developmental, cognitive, and emotional, as well as environmental (Kazdin, 1988a; Ronen, 1992, 1997b). The environmental approach views change of any kind as a stimulus that elicits stress and anxiety, which are then followed by behavior change or an increase in the number of symptoms (Kazdin, 1988a; Mash & Terdal, 1988).

Researchers agree that children develop symptoms and stress following a traumatic exposure. The debate mainly concerns the effect of the trauma. Some researchers believe the stress is short lived, and soon conceived as a challenge, in ways that can enhance development (Dubrow & Garbarino, 1988; Freud & Burlingham, 1943). Others view it as one that leaves permanent scars and evolves into posttraumatic stress disorder (Furman, 1986).

The Developmental Approach

While the first trend in the study of children's traumatic reactions focuses on environmental events (the kind of stressor and the outcome in presenting symptoms), the second trend focuses on developmental features. The developmental approach proposes that the specific child's response is mediated not by the kind of stressor, but rather by the child's current developmental phase. Development refers to the changing structure of behavior over the lifespan, indicating not only changing degrees of organism complexity, but also changes in the biological and psychological substructures emerging and unfolding in social surroundings (Shapiro, 1995).

Children are raised and educated by imitating and learning from their immediate surroundings. Up through elementary school age, due to their cognitive and emotional characteristics, children are more influenced by their immediate surroundings (i.e. family, immediate school environment) than by more distant events (e.g. in the community, in other homes) (Freud & Burlingham, 1943; Rahav & Ronen, 1994). Children 6–11 years old, in what Piaget (1924) called the concrete operational period, tend to be egocentric and to view concepts as related to their own experience. These youngsters tend to assess their experiences according to their moods, specific situations, and the people around them. Children this age find it difficult to understand concepts such as the finality of death, the likelihood of pain as a consequence of one's actions, relativity, or the perception of danger. They feel events within the close circle of the family to have a much greater impact, and even in times of disaster may be more influenced by family members' responses to the traumatic event than by their own perceptions of the catastrophe. Thus, whether or not the event is traumatic for the child depends on the way the child construed the event as traumatic.

Thus, the developmental trend highlights the child's developmental stage as the chief explanation for his or her behavior, in terms of age-appropriate responses and coping skills. Many child disturbances involve developmental considerations. Only through knowledge of normal developmental processes can one begin to understand deviations in development and their importance for assessment and intervention (Forehand & Weirson, 1993). It seems that an integration of the two approaches (environmental and developmental) is in order. While the developmental approach would submit that the responses of same-age children to various traumatic events can be similar, treatment considerations should take into account the sheer variety of personal, familial, social, natural, and manmade environmental traumatic experiences, and especially the unique characteristics of traumatic abuse by a parent or family member.

The Unique Case of Child Abuse

While facing an external traumatic event, the child is within the protective family he or she can rely on (such as earthquake, flood, or war). However, cases of abuse and neglect are usually incurred by the child's close environment. The child lives in the air of secrecy, communal denial, sense of guilt, and fear of rupturing the family unit by speaking out. Therefore, there is usually no one that abused children feel they can trust or depend on for help. Abuse is considered to be one of the most traumatic experiences to which a child can be exposed. Of the children referred to the U.S. social services between 1976 and 1982, 64% experienced "deprivation of necessities" (i.e. inadequate clothing, nutrition or medical care, exposure to hazards, or being left unattended), while 25% were the victims of physical abuse (e.g. bruised, cut, burned, or internally injured). Emotional and sexual abuse accounted for another 11% (Russell & Trainor, 1984).

Rapid cultural changes have been manifested in increasing societal awareness and responsibility to protect children from being harmed by their environment (Wolf, 1988).

Assessment

Regardless of the kind of trauma or the child's developmental stage, assessment of traumatized children is a complicated task necessitating multifarious assessment measures. McCloskey and Walker (2000) examined a sample of children exposed to chronic abuse and to various kinds of single-event trauma, using a structured diagnostic interview. Of the children reporting a traumatic event, 24.6% met the diagnostic criteria for posttraumatic stress disorder. Also, children with posttraumatic stress disorder displayed comorbidity across different symptom classes, most notably phobia and separation anxiety. Rasmussen (1999) added that assessment and treatment of sexually abused children is even more complicated, because of the shame, injury, and wish to hide the event from others and keep the secret in the family. A specific need exists to develop methods that carefully identify children who have been sexually abused and to formulate appropriate treatment plans.

Assessment of children's responses to various types of dangerous situations, trauma, and stress is strongly linked to their ability to understand, express, or cope with emotions. As described in Part I, in the course of development, children are increasingly able to demonstrate signs of emotions. This is manifested in their ability to talk about emotions, show a growing comprehension of emotional terms, understand situations that elicit emotions, induce emotions in themselves and others, understand emotional cues, and integrate successive or simultaneous emotions (Terwogt & Olthof, 1989). When negative affects are elicited as a result of parents' harmful actions toward their child, the ability for the child to develop a healthy emotional attachment with the parental figures is disrupted. Thus, a high likelihood exists for broader damage to the child's well being, and the possibilities for the child to learn appropriate emotional responding and to develop healthy experiences are at risk.

Treatment

The diversity in the type of traumatic events to which children are exposed complicates our ability to study, assess, and treat the traumatic disorder. Below, I will be presenting a case study of an abused child; therefore, I will relate this section to the treatment of traumatic responses to abuse and neglect.

Undertaking the treatment of children who suffer a traumatic reaction to experiences of neglect and abuse is a complex task that involves rendering changes in all areas of the child's life: behavior, emotions, and thoughts. None of these can be changed, however, as long as the child continues to be unsafe and unprotected. Therefore, therapists are obliged, first of all, to ascertain that the child becomes personally secure and protected in a safe environment, and only then, to start helping the child accept, cope, and overcome the traumatic events.

All of the various approaches to treating children who have undergone a traumatic abusive event share a common view espousing the dual need to involve the environment in treatment and to directly treat the traumatic child. In general, in cases of exposure to a natural or manmade traumatic event, an important part of treating traumatized children focuses on parents' supervision and parental therapy. Alexander (1999) emphasized that working with parents will facilitate their understanding of the impact of trauma on children and their familiarity with the normal responses children are likely to experience. In cases of child abuse, in particular, working with the environment is crucial. It is impossible to change the abused child's coping style without relating to the environment. Therefore, treatment of abused children usually includes the family. When the child had been abused by the father, the abusive father should be targeted to help decrease the abuse and teach him anger control, relaxation, and assertiveness skills (Gambrill, 1995a,b). Often, treatment of the child can only be achieved after the child's placement in a new environment, with the hope that this change will "do the job" (Kazdin, 1988a; Wolf, 1988). When the child is placed in a new home, involvement of the adoptive parents in a parent-training program will enhance parental competence and reduce stress (Gambrill, 1995b).

Prior et al. (1999) conducted interviews with foster care workers, residential caretakers, and social workers of children who experienced abuse and neglect, as well as with the children themselves. Their findings highlighted the following as essential features in professional intervention: emotional support and reassurance, provision of information and explanations, and arrangement and coordination of services including counseling or therapy. The findings of this study reinforce the need to refocus professionals' responses to abused children and their families.

No one single approach has been found efficient for treating traumatized children. The most common treatments are preventive methods for families at risk, parental supervision for reducing situational stress among high-risk families (Wolf, 1988), and community based intervention strategies, in addition to individual treatment of the child.

As mentioned before, while parents counseling and supervision are important, it is impossible to help the child overcome the traumatic abuse experience without direct individual therapy. This section will briefly describe three major therapeutic approaches that have been applied for individual treatment of traumatized abused children: psychodynamic therapy, cognitive behavioral therapy, and constructivist therapy.

Psychodynamic therapy. The psychodynamic treatment of traumatized children aims to allow them to become aware of those experiences that have been unmanageable. It is directed toward processing the traumatizing memories and reintegrating them into the child's world without being overwhelmed by terror (Rosie, 2000). Psychodynamic treatment can be conducted in an individual or group setting. Individual therapy follows the same basic rules of other psychodynamic treatment, which are usually applied through play therapy that helps the child express traumatic emotions and obtain insight into his or her situation. A unique kind of treatment is offered in group therapy. The group experience provides a setting that replaces the family role and permits the child's psychic and developmental wounds to receive some healing (Keyser et al., 2000). Family members are often unable to deal with the trauma constructively, giving either direct or indirect cues that talking about the painful event is unacceptable. Thus, the wounds continue to fester and development is blocked. The group offers a model for restoration of an ideal, caring "family" consisting of empathic adults (usually therapists) and other children who are accepting and understanding. Keyser and colleagues (2000) presented seven cases of children aged 7–9 who had experienced trauma and had been treated in this "family group." They described how the group created for these children a circle of people who could walk with them through the suffering, allowing them to verbalize their personal stories.

Cognitive behavior therapy. The cognitive behavioral treatment of traumatized children applies fear reduction techniques such as exposure, relaxation, and desensitization, as well as cognitive techniques such as cognitive restructuring and imagery training. Cohen et al. (2000) reviewed four major components of cognitive behavior therapy, which they view as central to the treatment of trauma in children: exposure, cognitive processing and reframing, stress management, and parental treatment. They concluded that, despite growing empirical support for the effectiveness of trauma-focused cognitive behavioral therapy in decreasing psychological symptomology, data on the relative contribution of the individual components remain inadequate.

Constructivist therapy. The implementation of constructivist therapy with traumatized children should be directed toward the child's own major metaphors and narratives, allowing the child to find new meaning in his or her personal experience and learning to open up rather than to close down as a result of the traumatic experiences. Knowledge on constructivist therapy with traumatic children continues to be limited. Constructivism emphasizes the need to find meaning for internal rather than external events, in keeping with the need to view the traumatic event through the child's own eyes (Ronen, 1996a). Therapists always strive to appreciate each client's subjective point of view (Neimeyer, 1995a,b), but for children this takes on stronger significance and is especially indicated in treating traumatized children.

While treating children who have suffered a traumatic event, the trauma cannot be avoided or changed. However, the way one processes it and deals with accompanying feelings of guilt, fear, and so on can have a critical impact on the ability to live a full and adaptive life following the traumatic experience (Ronen, 1996a; Swell, 1995). Central effort should be made, therefore, to enter the child's own world through empathic understanding. Instead of looking for facts, objective reality, or valid, reliable, external information, the therapist should attempt to gain a workable understanding of what the traumatic event means for the specific child (Neimeyer & Mahoney, 1995). As described in Part 1, therapists can use their own conceptual systems to learn to feel what the child feels, how the incident is perceived, what the child believes his or her reaction stands for, and how the child has detrimentally constructed his or her own reality. This attempt to step into the child's world can assist in determining how best to help the child reconstruct the traumatic event into another frame of reference.

Ronen (1996a) proposed a constructivist model for treating traumatized children. The model, comprising an adaptation of the SCIM described in Chapter 5 of this book, will be presented next in detail. The following case study describes the cognitive–constructivist therapy of an abused girl adopted during middle childhood. Therapy aimed to facilitate her development and empower her through the reinforcement of her positive abilities for change. The creative responsibility for change was shared between the therapist, who proposed new experiences such as metaphors, imagination, and role-play, and the child, who was expected to try them.

THE CASE OF LEE: ABUSE, NEGLECT, AND ADOPTION

Lee was 8 years old at the time of her referral to my clinic. She had been adopted one year earlier. At the time of the adoption, her adoptive parents began attending a parent-counseling group under my supervision. (This case was described in part in Ronen, 1998a). Her biological mother had died when Lee was age 5, after an extended period of heavy drug abuse. During the following two years of living with her biological father, Lee evidenced behavioral and emotional disorders, including sudden mood changes, regressive behaviors (crying, diurnal enuresis), fears, vomiting, hitting her peers, and disruptive behavior in the classroom. The social service agency discovered that her father was sexually abusing Lee. At the time of this revelation, Lee was questioned and interviewed by social workers, which enabled her to talk about what had happened to her. Lee was placed in a foster home while her father was tried in court, and she was helped to testify against him. Several months later, Lee's father was sentenced to prison, and she was put up for adoption. Her adoptive parents did not know how to deal with her anger and negativism; they felt helpless when she constantly rebelled and refused to accept their demonstrations of love. They decided to seek individual help beyond the group in which they were involved, and they came to me for consultation.

Intake Session with Lee's Adoptive Parents

Usually, I insist on meeting the parents and referred child together for the first session. The reason for this approach is that I am interested in learning how the child presents the problem, how the parents react to the child's presentation, and how the child responds to the parents' description of the problem. The family meeting enables me to gain information on communication discrepancies and relationships within the family, which are more difficult to ascertain while seeing each of them separately. However, in this case, I had already met Lee's parents in a parent group I conducted, and I knew how difficult the situation was and how disinclined Lee was to cooperate with the referral. I therefore invited her parents alone for a first intake session. This meeting centered on ascertaining the changes that had transpired in Lee's family since I last met with the parents, completing details on partial information at my disposal, and deciding about the optimal design for treatment.

Intake Session with Lee and Her Adoptive Parents

Next, I invited Lee together with her parents. This session was very important for me, because it enabled me to directly observe Lee's behavior. As they entered the room, the mother put her hand on Lee's shoulder. Immediately, Lee rushed forward into the room, to escape her mother's touch. She sat in the corner of the room, alone, on the edge of the sofa, with her head down. She did not initiate any conversation, and when asked if there was anything she wanted to add or relate, she just shrugged her shoulders and shook her head. She only spoke on several occasions during that meeting, when the father made comments about Lee being a smart, talented child or about how much they loved and cared about her. At these times, with a mocking facial expression, she burst out with replies like: "Oh, just quit it! I told you to stop all that nonsense!" When the parents told me about her disruptive behavior in class, she started yelling and told them they were lying, because she did not do those things. What impressed me most in that session was that this little girl, who could look very pretty, was extremely sad and angry, and that there was not the slightest glitter in her eyes nor any hint of laughter in her voice.

As I mentioned earlier, assessment begins the minute we first see the client. The way Lee sat down, the way she responded to her parents, and her sorrowful countenance provided very important cues contributing to my ability to assess her.

As delineated in Chapter 4, my selection of assessment methods for Lee was based on her age (see Table 4.3) and the nature of her problem, childhood trauma (see Table 4.2). Lee was in the stage of middle childhood, where she was occupied by a concrete operational way of thinking. At that age, assessment should be based on environmental reports from the teacher, parents, and even peers. However, at the age of 8, Lee could also be directly assessed, mainly by nonverbal, projective testing. In considering the nature of Lee's problem, her range of behavioral and emotional disorders cut across the board along all four types of referral to therapy (see an elaboration in Phase 2 below). Environmental reports would contribute mainly to learning about Lee's acting-out disorders and social problems, whereas her acting-in, emotional problems could best be evaluated by assessing Lee directly.

Thus, as described above, I interviewed the adoptive parents to learn about Lee's difficulties, and I also observed the family. In addition, I visited her school to observe her behavior with peers. I did not interview her classmates because I did not want her to feel embarrassed or singled out as an identified patient. However, in observing Lee's behavior, I saw that during recess she remained alone, did not join in the other children's activities, looked sad, and appeared on the verge of tears on several occasions. I talked with the teacher, and learned from her about Lee's disruptive behavior, but the teacher admitted that this did not seem to her as problematic as were Lee's loneliness and suffering. She interpreted the disruptive behavior as a bid for attention and said she could handle this and was able to get along with Lee. Environmental assessment underscored that Lee was a sad, suffering, lonely girl who seemed to be experiencing undue stress.

To enhance our understanding of Lee's emotional problems through direct testing, I invited Lee to an individual session with me.

First Session with Lee

Lee was well accustomed to being assessed, analyzed, and met by counselors, social workers, and therapists. At first, she sat down, saying, "So, you're another one of those, aren't you?" I answered, "I hope not," and she asked curiously, "How come?" I told her that I believe each of us is different and unique, with different preferences and interests. I said that my goal was to try and find the ways in which she was different and unique, and what she needed over and above anything else. She looked at me and said, "Well, we'll see." As her adoptive mother had mentioned, she sounded like an experienced old woman.

Lee looked around at pictures I had in the room and spontaneously made all kinds of negative remarks. About a painting of a lion and a rabbit she commented, "That lion will eat the rabbit up completely, nothing will be left. I know it. That rabbit's going to die." Looking at a poster of a man reaching his hand out to a boy, she asked, "Why doesn't he run away? That man will hit him."

In this first session, I asked Lee to draw a picture of a girl. When I saw the drawing, I almost cried. She said the picture was of a girl eating ice cream, but it seemed sadly clear to me that the girl had a penis in her mouth. She wrote a caption: "The girl who didn't take her hands out of her mouth."

As another projective assessment technique, we started playing some "I wish I were" games. I asked Lee, "If you weren't a girl but a color, what kind of color do you think you would be?" Without hesitation, Lee replied, "Black!" Then I asked her, "Now, if you were weather, what kind of weather would you be?" and Lee answered, "A great storm." When I asked her about a flower, she said, "A rose because it has thorns" and about a tree she said, "A prickly tree." As an animal, she hesitated between a snake and a lion, "The snake is bad and kills people, but the lion is a stronger animal. Everyone is afraid of a lion. But a lion is also the king and a pretty animal." In every metaphor, she emphasized the need to protect herself, to be able to harm others, and to keep others from touching her. Although expressing doubt about my ability to help her, Lee seemed to enjoy the attention in this first session and verbalized her agreement to meet with me regularly for therapy.

As I played association games with Lee, observed her behavior in the room during play, and listened to her own particular interpretations to the pictures on the walls, I was able to see, even at the beginning, Lee's preponderance of difficult, sad, suspicious, and other negative associations to the stimuli in her world. However, I was also impressed by her ability to observe little details and notice everything around her. Although she seemed troubled and sad, Lee demonstrated no problems concentrating and revealed a very good conversational ability. She used a very fluent, rich language and seemed to be very mature in her capability to analyze and understand things. It was very easy to talk with her, but I often found I had to remind myself how young she was.

Phase 1 of Decision Making: Does Lee Need Therapy or Not?

In determining whether Lee's presenting problem was deviant and whether or not her disorder warranted treatment, I considered the four main components described in Chapter 4 (Table 4.1). Relating to diagnostic criteria in the *DSM-IV* (American Psychiatric Association, 1994), Lee's behavior fit the criteria for post-traumatic behavior. Lee presented a large range of emotional and behavioral symptoms that could be the result of past trauma. The frequency of her behaviors did not change in her new surroundings. Her difficulties to trust others, to express emotion, and to socialize with others all seemed to pose a risk to her future, and later on might affect her ability to develop an independent identity. In terms of similarity to other children of her own age, sex, and culture, Lee's behavior was clearly deviant and did not resemble normal developmental disorders. She did not have social relationships that characterized her age.

With regard to family and child variables relating to motivation and support, Lee's adoptive parents evidenced great motivation to help her change, and were ready to support and help her in every necessary way. Lee herself did not show motivation for change. However, I did not expect her to be motivated, due to her past history. I was sure that, in time, as she learned to trust me and know me better, I would also be able to help her develop expectations for the future, thus facilitating her development of motivation for change.

The final consideration consisted of the ability to help Lee change. Although her past trauma could not be changed or eradicated, I believed that therapy was necessary and could help Lee develop better relationships with her adoptive family, a healthier acceptance of herself, and improved peer relationships. The foregoing criteria, therefore, pointed clearly to the need to treat Lee.

Phase 2 of Decision Making: Classifying Lee's Referral and Goals for Change

The second phase of decision making concerned assessing Lee's referral and establishing treatment goals in relation to the therapeutic goals and developmental tasks defined in Chapter 4. Looking at Lee's disorders in light of the four main goals of child therapy (increasing behavior, decreasing behavior, removing anxiety, and facilitating development; see Table 4.2), it can be seen that Lee suffered from all of the possible problems. She exhibited problems characterized as undercontrolled, acting-out disorders that needed to be decreased. These included her anger, shouting, hitting, and disruptive classroom behavior. Her social skills, loneliness, suspiciousness, and difficulties in trusting others were problems related to overcontrolled emotional disorders, pinpointing behaviors that needed to be increased. Lee also presented anxious behavior combined with fears, crying, and vomiting symptoms, reflecting the third type of goal, the need to remove anxiety. There were also behaviors that related to the fourth goal, facilitating development. In middle childhood, Lee was at the stage where she must cultivate a personal identity and self-control. Her past trauma had caused inhibitions and the lack of an ability to develop trusting, mature relationships with adults and with peers. It seemed, therefore, that Lee needed to be helped in every possible way, to achieve changes targeting all four of the main goals in children's therapy.

In terms of the developmental tasks facing Lee, at this age she faced two main social roles. One, she should develop the self-control skills necessary to participate appropriately and obediently in her school and home environments, and to be able to function independently. Two, she should develop her own self-identity, which would continue to unfold over adolescence. Lee's past trauma had affected her by damaging both areas of functioning. As a result of being abused, she found it difficult to master self-control skills, and she had acquired fears, anxieties, mistrust, and suspiciousness.

The therapeutic goals and developmental tasks considered in this phase emphasized the need for Lee's treatment to focus on imparting her with the skills and resources necessary to cope with her future life. Also, she avoided developmentally normal behavior that characterized other children her age. She needed help to develop loving, caring relationships with others and with herself. Her treatment would also necessarily focus on helping Lee establish self-trust, self-acceptance, and the capacity to cope with her anxieties and fears.

Phase 3 of Decision Making: Selecting Who Should Be Treated

Both Lee's developmental stage and the nature of her problem accentuated the need to select an individual treatment setting for her. During middle childhood (see Table 4.4), children have the necessary cognitive skills to conduct meaningful conversation and can enjoy individual therapy. Lee exhibited acting-out disorders suggesting the need to continue working with Lee's parents and possibly with her teacher on issues relating to discipline. Those disorders can best be treated by supervising the environment (see Table 4.5). However, the insufficiency of past parent counseling to render a change implied that Lee needed to first undergo some changes in herself and in accepting her new environment, in order for that environment to effectively reinforce her positive behavior and help eliminate her undesired conduct.

Clearly, Lee also exhibited an assortment of emotional disorders. Such disorders are very difficult to treat in the presence of the parents, especially adoptive parents with whom a trusting bond had not yet evolved.

For several reasons, it seemed to me that family therapy was contraindicated. Lee's biological father was incarcerated and already receiving treatment at the prison facility. Her adoptive parents had already participated in a parents' group, and Lee herself appeared to be at high risk and as yet unready to develop a new healthy relationship with her adoptive parents. Therefore, we decided that I would begin by individually treating Lee while meeting her parents and teacher when needed. As she progressed, we would consider family intervention.

Phase 4 of Decision Making: Selecting Lee's Optimal Treatment Modes

In designing the most appropriate techniques for change in Lee's treatment, my guidelines (in Chapter 4) proposed that a number of therapist, child, developmental, and problem variables be considered. With regard to therapist variables, I felt that treating Lee would be a challenge for me as a therapist. It was difficult to listen to her rigid negative verbalizations about the world, other people, and the future. In addition, it would be a challenge to understand the diversity and paradoxical trends in her behavior.

With respect to child variables, I considered Lee's motivation as well as her individual hobbies and preferences, necessitating the selection of methods that would best suit her way of thinking and interests. Although rebellious toward her adoptive parents, Lee sought out attention and, as therapy started, seemed to be ready to cooperate with me. In addition, like most girls her age, she enjoyed playing with dolls, and loved drawing. As therapy progressed, I found out that Lee loved music very much. She spent a great deal of her day listening to the radio and watching television clips of new songs, and she was able to sing the songs with all the words. This proclivity toward music could certainly be used in therapy as a way to increase her motivation for collaboration and as a frame of reference for successful behavior while working on self-esteem issues. These communication modes were conducive to an interesting integration of verbal and nonverbal therapeutic processes.

In terms of Lee's developmental stage, in middle childhood both direct and indirect therapy can be applied. Lee was already at the stage where she could talk about problems, but the use of nonverbal therapy continues to be very common at this age (see Table 4.6). Moreover, the types of problems presented by Lee comprised a mixture of behavioral and emotional disorders. The latter are usually easier to address via nonverbal, indirect therapy (see Table 4.7).

In contemplating all of these considerations, I found myself spending many hours deliberating about which techniques and modes I should implement in Lee's therapy, in which sequence, so as to help her overcome her terrible past and enjoy her improved present and future. Finally, I decided to use cognitive–constructivist psychotherapy for teaching her self-control skills, utilizing creative methods to help foster her ability to open up to emotional responses. The use of creative methods such as narratives, storytelling, imagery, music, and drawing were introduced to lessen her sense of helplessness, weakness, and difficulty when talking about her past. She felt very confident, resourceful, and successful while drawing, writing, singing, and reading, in contrast with the feelings of unwillingness, closedness, and suspicion she revealed when asked to talk about her past. I expected that by using tools and modes with which she felt safe, I could empower her to develop assurance in areas where she did not feel so secure. However, in view of Lee's intelligence and verbal ability, I integrated all of these creative techniques into verbal therapy.

Under the umbrella of cognitive–constructivist therapy, a major focus of therapy would be Lee's abuse and trauma. I decided I should target therapy toward three main aims (Ronen, 1996a). The first aim involved the immediate experience of the trauma. An important goal of therapy was to help Lee change her attitude toward the traumatic event. She had to learn to accept that traumatic events had been experienced. She could not forget or erase her past; however, she could be helped to learn to live with it. She had to free herself of the sense of guilt and responsibility she felt for those traumatic events. She also had to be encouraged to become aware of the thoughts, emotions, and behaviors that her traumatic past elicited, and to allow herself to express them. In addition, Lee required guidance in trying both to live with these and to understand that in time these feelings could be changed. The second aim involved changing the meaning (i.e. the construction) of the event in order to cope with it more effectively. The third aim was directed toward the future, helping her to grow out of the traumatic experience and empowering her to be open to the world and give other experiences a chance, as a first step toward building a healthy relationship with her new family (Ronen, 1998a).

Treatment with Lee

I treated Lee using my basic self-control model (SCIM) comprising four intervention modules (see Table 5.1). This model was adapted specifically to traumatized children (Ronen, 1996a). The application of the SCIM to the area of responses to trauma necessitated an adaptation of two modules. First, in the initial reframing module, particular effort would be invested in helping Lee learn to accept that her past trauma could not be changed or forgotten. In contrast to cases of anxieties and fears, where children must learn to take personal responsibility and learn to overcome and eliminate their problems, Lee must learn to avoid blaming herself and to develop more accepting ways to live with that past. This first module would encompass a virtual key to unlocking Lee's treatment success. The second adaptation comprised the placement of greater emphasis on Lee's emotional expression; in the third, attentional focus module, she would need particular help in learning to identify internal events, thoughts, and feelings without trepidation and in becoming able to live with those affects related to her past. Instead of focusing on increasing awareness the focus is on learning to accept and let go.

SCIM module 1: Cognitive restructuring and redefinition. Usually, the first module is based on teaching the child to accept responsibility for his or her behavior. However, with traumatic abuse, the child needs to learn that he or she was not responsible for the abuse. It was not her fault. Children are raised to obey their parents, and she did what every other child would have done. She did nothing wrong! What happened was her father's fault and responsibility, not hers (Ronen, 1996a, 1998a). Therapy aimed to achieve this goal through doll playing, with a focus on understanding what the doll felt. At first she played with the dolls, allowing herself to talk about what happened, to yell and to cry. Then, I encouraged her to differentiate between what parents usually do and what her father did. I wanted to give Lee a safe foundation for developing a healthy relationship with her adoptive parents ("Your biological father did wrong. Most fathers don't act that way. Your adoptive father is different"). I tried to help her redefine her life as two different entities: the little Lee who lived with a father who harmed her, and the older Lee who is lucky to have protective, loving parents. She needed to learn the difference between the two families and feel safe enough in her present life. This step took a long time to achieve. Throughout the whole process of treatment, we came back to it again and again, as she was looking for assurance and confidence, examining her present life over and over again.

I decided to use imagery techniques with Lee for many reasons. One, as Lazarus (1984) proposed, imagery presents the hidden powers of the mind. An image is a mental picture of something not actually present. By using imagination, it is possible to reach out to many realities that are physically absent, as in playing both sides of a chess game in one's head. There are definite differences in people's capacity to form clear vivid images. Some individuals can conjure up perfectly distinct images that are as clear as the actual event. Others possess very clear (but not perfect) images (Lazarus, 1984). Lee's abuse transpired in the past, when she was still very young, and she demonstrated difficulty in remembering details. However, we could not continue working without helping her recall and express as many as possible of these fearful traumatic experiences. Another reason for selecting imagery was Lee's intense difficulty in discussing her experiences of sexual abuse. She objected to the idea of even referring to them. However, the use of imagery can often bypass verbal roadblocks and get to the root of the matter. Many people tend to overintellectualize, confusing themselves and everybody else with verbiage. Imagery methods can permit a therapist to sidestep these barriers (Lazarus, 1984).

At first we used imagery to elicit her early memories, as a basis for trying to accept and understand the little Lee. We continued using creative imagination even as she progressed, because imagery not only emphasizes what has happened in the past but also has a healing power by pinpointing change. I asked Lee to imagine two different Lees: the safe 8-year-old Lee and the young abused 5-year-old. I asked her to visually observe the differences in the way they act, their appearance, the way they talk, and the expressions on their faces. Then she was asked to draw the two Lees. At the beginning of treatment, young Lee was drawn like a monster in black, with a big mouth and long hands, whereas "big Lee" was very pale, thin, and vague. As the treatment progressed, I asked her once again to check if she still felt the same way. This time, she changed the figures. The young Lee was drawn as much smaller, whereas the older Lee had become a much bigger figure. I also asked her to portray herself in the future, and she drew a large, brightly colored figure. Lee still felt frightened by the idea of a brighter future, offering the reservation, "Well, this isn't exactly what I feel now, but I think that it's what I'll feel one day after we finish therapy!" As she felt more secure visualizing the young, abused girl, I asked her to imagine herself talking to and comforting the abused 5-year-old Lee, accepting and forgiving her, and telling her that the older Lee was very different and therefore could say goodbye to the young one.

These imagination exercises were very difficult for Lee. It was easy for her to use the imagery, but she would feel herself becoming a part of the picture so quickly that she would easily begin sobbing or shouting and once even tried to hit herself. The first two months of treatment sessions involved much crying, yelling, and aggression. Both of us would end these sessions exhausted. Still, I thought it was important for her to let her emotions out, especially considering that her adoptive parents were afraid to let her do so and would begin reassuring and calming her whenever she mentioned abusive events from her past.

During the first several weeks of treatment, Lee became angry whenever I tried to talk with her about replacing her negative automatic thoughts with other, mediated ones. Gradually, through a process combining drawing, playing, and Socratic questioning, Lee started accepting the idea that as a child she had been helpless. She even became ready to begin talking about self-forgiveness. She reached the point where she could say: "But I will not be helpless anymore. I'm learning judo." At this stage, we could start working toward different goals.

SCIM module 2: Problem analysis. In the second module of self-control treatment, we tried to learn to identify the process characterizing how she thought and felt about her past. This phase is very similar to the original SCIM. We emphasized the analysis of the links between emotions, thoughts, and behaviors, and attempted to change her automatic negative thoughts into mediated ones. These processes were implemented by using illustrations to exemplify how the brain commands the body and by employing games where I "commanded" Lee to do things and watched how she accomplished them. We tried to understand and explain her negative attitudes towards her adoptive parents, focusing on Lee's acting-out behavior as an outcome of her fears of loving them and then being disappointed. We practiced changing her automatic negative thoughts into mediated ones; for example, taking the thought "I shouldn't get close to them," which elicited rejection and avoidance behavior, and transforming it into another way of thinking: "Maybe I can try to be nice to them and see what happens."

SCIM module 3: Attentional focus. Another change in the SCIM for traumatic children can be found in the third module, that of attentional focus. In every other form of treatment, it is important to focus on increasing sensitivity to internal stimuli. In cases of trauma, in addition to increasing awareness, there is also a need to decrease sensitization, learning to accept and live with. It is also important to emphasize learning to express positive as well as negative emotions, and learning to live with some feelings of past distress and anger. This module targeted Lee's feelings, which she had been avoiding and ignoring. We tried to identify different kinds of emotions such as fear, anxiety, stress, and anger. At first, she was not ready to talk about positive emotions, but gradually she agreed to start exercises on happiness, joy, and so on. We attempted to pinpoint the place in her body where she felt sensations (her stomach when she's afraid) and the kind of sensations (contractions), learning that internal signs exist for every feeling. Lee was taught to draw a ladder and rate the intensity of the emotion she felt by climbing the ladder. She received a homework assignment to record one emotion every day: its location in the body and its intensity. Lee found it very hard to talk about emotion and at first rejected this task. At that time, she had a birthday and received a camera from her parents. I decided to use her new hobby to facilitate our work in this area. I asked her first to take photographs of strangers in the street and to bring them to the sessions. We then observed them, trying to guess their emotions by looking at external signs (serious, smiling, angry). Then, she offered to take pictures of her own parents, and at last even brought a picture of herself, saying: "This is the happy Lee. You know why I was happy? It was my birthday party for my friends."

SCIM module 4: Self-control exercises. In the fourth module, Lee practiced tasks such as using positive imagery to overcome her traumatic memories and to construct a new picture of a positive future. Relaxation before going to sleep, self-recording, self-talk, and changing automatic thoughts to mediated thoughts constituted this phase of treatment.

Using the metaphor of an architect, she was encouraged to design the way she wished to see her new life, new friends, and new family, attempting to overcome the fears of letting herself feel positive emotions and then be disappointed and cast aside again. Through narrative and storytelling methods, she learned to accept her feelings, to expose herself to the memories, and to let them go.

The end of the first year of treatment was based on storytelling.

Lee was asked to pretend as if she was giving a book proposal to a publisher and needed to write down all the chapters that would be included in it. The book was to be about her own life. This technique was suggested by Neimeyer (1995) for enhancing self-understanding of one's own personal meaning-making by viewing the way one relates to one's life as a list of chapters. Neimeyer developed questions to accompany the technique, such as: "Who else could write your book? Who wouldn't you like to write your book? How would your book look different if someone else had written it?" We observed the kind of language Lee used (passive or active), the names of the chapters, and the process she described (chronological versus event-linked; the person versus the environment; Ronen & Rosenbaum, 1998). An interesting sign of change was revealed by the names Lee gave to her chapters:

1. The Happy Family (describing her birth and the first years with both parents together)
2. The Poor Girl Who has a Sick Mother (relating to her mother during the process of dying)
3. The Cruel Father
4. The Wish to Run Away

As difficult as it was to see those names, it was clear that Lee did not take the blame on herself any longer. She had stopped seeing herself as the cause and the reason for her problems, but rather saw herself as a victim of events.

The exciting part was when I asked her to continue her book and write the names of the future chapters, and Lee added:

5. The Girl who Could Not Accept Her Parents' Love
6. Starting to Love the Family
7. The Wonderful Mother

When Lee was asked to explain, she said she knew that right now she could not love her new parents, but she knew they were good, and she planned (in Chapter 6) to "start loving them" in a year. She explained that Chapter 7 would be her after she got married, when she would become the most wonderful mother one could be.

Phase 5 of Decision Making: Evaluating Lee at the End of Therapy and Maintaining Treatment Outcomes

Evaluation. The best way to evaluate the client's condition at the end of therapy is to return to the baseline assessments and compare baseline data to those at the end of therapy. At the onset of therapy, assessment was conducted via Lee's teacher, her parents, and Lee herself. Evaluation should also take into consideration treatment goals, which included removing anxiety, stress, and posttraumatic behavior, and helping Lee establish healthier skills for accepting herself and her parents (see Table 4.8). As mentioned before, in relation to Lee's developmental stage, in middle childhood, Lee should be evaluated via her parents' report, her own report, and direct observation of her behavior.

The parents' report emphasized the many changes Lee had undergone. They said that Lee was not as negative as she used to be, and she had become much more obedient. They could talk with her without constantly receiving the cynical, bitter answers she had given in the past, and they noted that it was easier to have friendly conservation with Lee. They also reported that most of her emotional symptoms (crying, sadness, loneliness) had disappeared. The mother said that when she touched her daughter, Lee no longer pushed her hands away or objected, although they had not yet initiated closer contact (hugs and kisses).

An interview with Lee's teacher also emphasized significant changes. As mentioned before, the teacher, even in the baseline interview, said she could handle Lee's disruptiveness. Now, she told me the disruptive behavior had substantially decreased, and most of Lee's present disruptions stemmed from her talking with other children during lessons. The teacher added that, as long as these conversations were quiet, she did not interfere, because she was happy to see Lee starting to establish social relations. The teacher also reported that Lee had begun to try to get involved in classroom activities and that she seemed to be happier. Lee did not initiate social activities, but when the class met to do things together (such as going to a movie or party), Lee would join them. During recess, she would go outside instead of staying in the class, and she would join other children. She had two close friends with whom she seemed to feel more comfortable, and though she appeared to feel less at ease in large crowds, Lee was not avoiding them.

Lee herself reported that she was not feeling as frightened as before, and she was almost not anxious. She said she thought she was having dreams now, but could not recall them. She no longer had nightmares or crying spells. She mentioned that she had begun talking to a few classmates at school. She said she would not call herself "very happy" but was no longer sad. While talking about her friends, she said she had two friends, and she thought two were enough and did not want any more.

Maintenance. After this evaluation at the end of one year of intensive therapy, it seemed that the time had arrived to "change gears" and shift to a maintenance stage of intervention. Due to Lee's wide range of problems, the severity of her disorders, and her history of abusive, neglectful relationships with adults, she needed a longer, more gradual separation from the therapist. We entered into a contract for an undetermined follow-up period where we would continue to meet once every two to three weeks. Lee was instructed to generalize her new ability to express positive emotion, initiate social contact, and participate in social events on her own, gradually transferring these newly learned skills and attitudes to her adoptive parents, her biological father, and her peers.

I do not know if anyone can resolve the problem of traumatic abusive experiences through treatment, whether it lasts one year, three, or ten. What I can say is that, at the present time, after one year of intensive treatment, and several months of follow-up sessions with Lee and her parents, Lee has started overcoming her behavior disorders and her negativity in her relationship with her parents. She is still occupied with her past memories, but she started developing more affective relationships with her new family. However, she does not see the world only as a place of war, fear, and injury; and some smiles and positive emotions have broken through, in increasing intensity. The way is still long, and we have much to accomplish. However, it seems that this year of individual therapy has provided the groundwork for family therapy in the near future, where we will be able to concentrate on constructing a healthy relationship for Lee within her new family.

This morning, as I was editing this chapter for the last time, I received a telephone call from the mother. She called me, very excited, because she wanted to share with me the experience she had during that last week, when Lee, for the first time, hugged her, kissed her, and told her she loved her. The mother said that Lee was also very nice to her father, and let him hug her, but she would not yet initiate touching him. Moreover, the mother said that, at this point, they were already certain that it was only a matter of time and patience until they reached the place they desired, normal loving relationships within the family.

9

Psychosomatic Pain

LITERATURE REVIEW

Pediatricians and psychologists have long recognized the relationship between physical and psychological factors in children's health. These relationships can be reflected in various diagnoses such as psychosomatic disorders or somatoform disorders, or the separate diagnosis of pain disorder. Siegel and Richards (1978) proposed the name somatic disorder to refer to any bodily dysfunction, irrespective of the presumed etiology, and avoided the distinction between "psychosomatic disorders" and other health related disorders.

The *DSM-IV* (American Psychiatric Association, 1994) relates to somatoform disorders among adults as the presence of physical symptoms that suggest a general medical condition and that are not fully explained by a general medical condition. The disorder includes somatization disorders, somatoform disorders, conversion disorder, pain disorder, hypochondriasis, and bodily dysomorphic disorders. It is defined as a history of many complaints beginning before the age of 30 years, and holds the following criteria: existence of at least four pain symptoms; two gastrointestinal symptoms other than pain; one sexual symptom, and one pseudoneurological symptom.

Psychosomatic disorders have been described as physical problems caused by emotional disturbance (Roberts, 1986). Psychosomatic disorder includes physical symptoms produced by psychological problems or stress such as asthma, vomiting, recurrent pain, and ulcerative colitis. It also includes physical problems caused or maintained by a faulty learning history or developmental anomalies such as encopresis, enuresis, psychogenic seizures, or tracheotomy addiction. In addition, it includes psychological problems associated with or following medical disorders, such as noncompliance to medical regimens and psychological maladjustment to chronic pain (Wright, 1977).

Studies related to somatoform disorders among children and adolescents have shown a high rate of frequency, comorbidity, and psychosocial impairment. Several recent studies investigated the frequency of somatoform disorders. In a survey of 1035 randomly selected students aged 12–17(Essau et al., 1999), about 13.1% met the *DSM-IV* mental disorders criteria for any somatoform disorder (American Psychiatric Association, 1994). Also, significantly more girls than boys were found to be affected by such disorders. Pain and conversion disorders were the most common type of somatoform disorders reported. The most common symptoms were headache, lump in the throat, and abdominal pain (Essau et al., 1999). In another random survey of 3021 adolescents, 50% were found as having suffered from one somatoform symptom at least once in their life (Lieb et al., 1998). The prevalence of somatoform disorders of any type was 13%. This study emphasized a high comorbidity with other disorders, which increased with age and was, moreover, associated with impairments in social skills. In a survey in the city of Florence, the one-year prevalence figures were as follows: 0.7% body dysmorphic disorder, 4.5% hypochondriasis, 0.6% somatoform pain disorder, 0.3% conversion disorder, 0.7% somatization disorder, and 13.8% undifferentiated somatoform disorder (Faravelli et al., 1997).

A separate and most difficult diagnosis to treat is the existence of pain in children. Varni and colleagues (1982) described four types of pain in children: pain resulting from a disease, pain resulting from injury or trauma, pain resulting from medical or dental procedures, and pain with no association to disease or injury. Fordyce (1976) suggested that some pains are environmentally influenced by reinforcements such as parental attention, a release from school, etc.

Only scant empirical evidence exists to support treatment approaches to pain and other somatoform disorders relating to children, with most interventions applied in accordance with clinical empirical considerations (Fritz et al., 1997).

Four main models address this disorder.

The stress model. According to this model, noxious or stressful stimuli result in increasing physiological activity which, if prolonged, can lead to lowered resistance of the body system and eventually to disease (Siegel & Smith, 1991). A major research focus in recent years has involved the effect of stressful life events on health related problems. It has been proposed that life changes, whether positive or negative, require some readjustment by the person affected. A consequence of frequent life-changing events is an enhanced susceptibility to disease. This model emphasizes the importance of personal resources (coping behaviors) and social support (Lazarus, 1966, Siegel & Smith, 1991). Therapy focuses on stress inoculation, which fosters coping skills and mobilizes social and family support.

The family system model. Various theories have addressed the role of the family in the etiology and maintenance of physical symptoms among its members. Particular concern has been focused on the nature of the family interaction patterns, regarding the somatic symptoms as playing a function in stabilizing and maintaining the status quo of the family system (Haggerty, 1983). Minuchin and his colleagues (Minuchin et al., 1975, 1978) suggested that families of children diagnosed as "psychosomatic" demonstrated a number of consistent characteristics, particularly when threatened by stresses. Such children were shown to be rigid in their rules and expectancies, to lack appropriate problem-solving skills, and to be overprotected. Intervention, therefore, was designed to change the dysfunctional patterns within the family's organization and interactions.

The behavioral model. Learning has been shown to play a significant role in a variety of somatic disorders. Automatic and visceral responses can be affected or altered by both respondent conditioning and operant conditioning. Somatic symptoms are regarded as the result of interactions between stress reactions and operant and respondent conditioning. The child develops pain either by observing and modeling painful behaviors of adults or by receiving considerable adult attention and comfort when reporting pain (Siegel & Smith, 1991). Therapy involves changing the consequences of the child's complaints, removing attention from undesired behavior, and increasing the rewards for desirable behavior.

The cognitive–perceptual model. This model examines the role of perceptual processes in the development of physical symptoms, emphasizing that a preoccupation with or heightened sensitivity to bodily states contributes to symptom development (Siegel & Smith, 1991). Pennebaker and Skelton (1978) suggested that attending to one's internal states serves to enhance the perceived intensity of physical symptoms. Persons who tend to focus on normal bodily sensations tend to report more symptoms. They exhibit a tendency to experience normal sensations as disturbing and respond to such sensations with hypervigilance. As a result, these sensations are amplified and misinterpreted. Treatment focuses on cognitive– behavioral techniques that emphasize one's cognitions and appraisals. Therapy should establish the context and meaning of the pain, emphasizing the link between life events and pain complaints (Varni et al., 1982). Children and parents are directed to keep incident records or diaries, to learn to trace the antecedents–behavior–consequences relationship (Roberts, 1986). The treatment accentuates helping families focus on the ways in which the child might deal appropriately with the pain when it occurs and how the child can maintain regular activities around it.

Most of these models have recommended that therapists conduct a psychosocial assessment with the child and the parents, as well as direct observation. An important and necessary part of treatment constitutes the parents, who should be taught that the problem is not "only in the child's head;" the child does suffer and needs help, and psychosomatic pains can be as harmful as every other pain. Redefinitions such as "behavioral habits" or "reactions to stress" often help (Roberts, 1986).

The next case study illustrates treatment of a child who suffered from psychosomatic and pain disorders.

DAN, A BOY WITH PSYCHOSOMATIC ACHES

One of my biggest surprises in an intake session was meeting Dan and his family. In a previous telephone call with his mother while trying to schedule an appointment, she told me about her gentle, delicate 11-year-old boy, who suffered from severe stomachaches accompanied by a feeling of nausea and the urge to vomit. Dan had been in and out of the hospital during the last year and a half; he had undergone all kinds of medical examinations to rule out a tumor, ulcer, or other medical problems. Following these aversive tests, it was decided that nothing was physically wrong with him, and that his symptoms were a response to stress. The doctors had recommended trying to find out whether he was anxious or suffering from stress or fears, which may be resulting in somatic pains.

Hearing the mother's description, I was expecting a thin, pale, delicate boy. I was surprised to see this tall, handsome, well-built child enter the room. Dan was noisy, full of humor, and repeatedly interrupted the conversation impatiently, having something to say about everything and everyone, usually joking cynically. At first sight, I thought I had confused Dan with another new referral from that same time, and I replaced his story of pain in my mind with that of another boy. It took me a while to realize that Dan was the boy suffering from somatic symptomology, and that it was my prejudice and preliminary wrong assumptions that made me react the way I did. How easy it is for us therapists, who seem to be open minded and flexible, to fall into rigid categorizations of our clients, and how terrible it is to think that I too was falling into that trap.

Unfortunately, that was not the only trap I fell into with Dan. I believed that suffering as much as he did, undergoing such strong stress, probably meant he had some severe disturbance that I would need to teach him how to control and that he needed to learn how to overcome his pain. I also held two other false assumptions: I conjectured that either he was a perfectionist, with overly high self-expectations and difficulties in fulfilling them, or else he had very pressuring, overly demanding parents who were responsible for the stress. Neither of these turned out to be the case.

Intake Session

The most important thing I was learning during the intake session was to be careful not to assume too many things too fast, to stay open minded, and to avoid diagnosis. The only way I could figure out what was happening was by staying open minded, listening, and letting the information in without trying to assess it.

Dan was the only child of two parents who emigrated from the Netherlands. He was born in Israel, and looked and behaved Israeli. He tried to avoid any signs of his parents being foreigners. Both of the parents were musicians. His mother was a pianist and worked as a piano teacher, and his father played the violin, teaching music in a school for the arts.

Both parents had adjusted well to Israeli society, had many friends, and enjoyed their life and their son. They could not have more children due to some medical problems of the mother. The two of them tried to give their child whatever he needed and devoted much time to him but did not spoil him. They were a loving couple, enjoyed traveling together, used to entertain a great deal and go out a lot, but also took care to spend time with their son and do things with him.

As a child, Dan was educated by his parents to be polite, gentle, and refrain from violence. However, as he grew, they realized that he was becoming frightened too easily. They decided to send him to self-defense courses, where he was trained in judo and karate. They tried to teach him to defend himself but not to start a fight unless absolutely necessary.

An important issue I was aware of concerned Dan's relationship with his parents. Dan would become angry whenever he thought other people could identify any sign whatsoever that his family was foreign, educated, or rich. He had changed his family name from that of his parents, using a different, more Israeli last name because he did not want any reminders of being a foreigner. He refused to talk Dutch and laughed at his parents' accent. Dan said he was ashamed of his parents' career as musicians. He wanted them to be "normal," so he told his friends his mother was a secretary and his father a teacher. He would not listen to classical music or go with them to concerts. He was angry whenever they spent money; he asked them to trade in their big fancy car for a modest, small one. He did not want to take or spend money and refused to wear new clothes. He called his parents by their first names, not "Mom" or "Dad." Dan told me about all this in a kind of cynical voice. His parents, on the other hand, were mostly passive and accepting about his attitudes toward them, their career and wealth, shrugging their shoulders as if to say: "That's what he wants. There's nothing we can do but accept it."

Another strong impression was related to Dan's manners. Dan seemed to be an extremely clever boy, with a strong sense of humor. He joked about everything and everyone, taking the role of a clown at times, but often turning his humor toward himself, as well. He talked a lot and seemed to be in control of himself and the environment (e.g. he decided when it was his parents' turn to talk, or when he wanted them to keep quiet). Yet, in contrast with his evident talents and strengths, Dan appeared very anxious about his social position, his relationships with other children, and his ability to cope during difficult situations with peers.

At the same time, I realized that Dan was really suffering physically. During the session, it was clear that he was in pain. Often, he held his stomach, bending over or changing his position while his face changed color. I could tell he was suffering. I thought he seemed too sensitive and overly aware of his internal cues and stimuli. He appeared to notice every change, feeling, or sensation in his body, and was concentrating too much on what was going on inside him.

Dan refused to accept the diagnosis of psychosomatic pain, crying and complaining that he was in pain and refusing to go to school because of how badly he felt.

As outlined in Chapter 4, the selection of reliable and valid tools for assessment required that I consider Dan's age (see Table 4.3) and the nature of his problem (see Table 4.2). Middle childhood is a stage when direct assessment methods can be applied. Based on the overcontrolled, emotional, and acting-in behaviors that Dan presented (see Phase 2 below), the best assessment method could be his own direct self-observation of complaints and self-rating of pain. Due to Dan's ability to talk about and describe his pain, I did not see any reason to give him empirical-emotional tests. Another important assessment tool comprised parental reports on Dan's school attendance and social activities. In view of the fact that Dan's problem related mostly to himself and his family, there was no reason to interview the teacher. Therefore, assessment was based on parents' interview and chiefly on observing Dan's behavior, as described below.

Phase 1 of Decision Making: Does Dan Need Therapy or Not?

As presented in the first part of the book, therapy should start with a continuing process of decision making. The first decision a therapist should make is whether or not the child needs therapy. Four main variables can help in making this decision (see Table 4.1). With regard to problem variables, Dan's complaints needed to be compared with common diagnostic criteria. No specific definition of psychosomatic disorder as a children's disorder is provided in the *DSM-IV* (American Psychiatric Association, 1994). However, according to the criteria found in the *DSM-IV* for adult psychosomatic disorder, Dan evidenced more than the required four psychosomatic complaints, suffered from various symptoms in addition to his pain, and exhibited these difficulties for longer than a year. The sexual symptom criterion was inappropriate for assessing a child. Nevertheless, sufficient data indicated that Dan fulfilled the criteria for somatoform disorder, thereby highlighting the risk posed to Dan's future if he were not treated.

In terms of developmental variables influencing the decision of whether or not therapy was warranted, most children of Dan's age are occupied with social relationships and do not pay much attention to aches, pains, or other physical symptoms. The extent of his complaints deviated from the norms for Dan's age, sex (girls more frequently report pain than do boys), and culture. Dan's overinvolvement with his bodily sensations, pains, and symptoms could clearly be considered deviant.

With respect to child and family variables, both Dan and his parents were very motivated for change. Dan was eager to get rid of his pain, and the parents were very worried about his condition. They were ready to comply with the treatment assignments and to support Dan in the process of trying to overcome his emotional as well as physical condition.

The fourth variable relates to prognosis. As mentioned above, adequate knowledge is unavailable on the efficacy of treatments for psychosomatic disorders. However, sufficient evidence exists to indicate that pain and somatoform disorders can be changed. Careful assessment, family support, and training in cognitive and behavioral techniques may be considered crucial components in the process of recovery (Roberts, 1986).

Assessment of all four variables contributing to the first phase of decision making clearly indicated that Dan required treatment, and that therapy would likely help him overcome, or at least minimize, his pain. Now that I had determined that Dan was in need of therapy, I could attempt to ascertain the kind of problems he suffered from at the time of referral and which goals therapy should target based on his behavior and its consequences.

Phase 2 of Decision Making: Classifying Dan's Referral and Goals for Change

As emphasized before, the treatment process combines nonstop decision making. The second phase of decision making relates to the reasons for referral, goals of treatment, and developmental tasks (see Tables 4.2 and 4.3). Of the four main kinds of disorders usually involved in children's referrals, Dan's therapy needed to focus on two: increasing behavior and removing anxiety. First, Dan needed to increase his social behavior. The literature often relates psychosomatic disorders to a lack of social skills. Looking at Dan's behavior problems, only very rarely did his psychosomatic complaints appear over weekends or holidays. Mostly, they appeared when Dan was encountering social activities such as going to school, extracurricular pastimes, or parties. Dan seemed to feel a strong need to be accepted by peers and also a fear of being different than others. In addition, in his old school, he had undergone some negative experiences where some children hit him, and he feared hurting them back. He had developed an avoidance reaction and had coped with this unpleasant social situation by developing pain and staying at home, which, in turn, only increased his apprehension of social contact. However, these symptoms comprised neither a social phobia nor a fear of social relationships. It was therefore important to teach Dan social skills that would foster his social behavior, increasing his self-confidence and self-acceptance.

The second goal was to remove anxiety and teach Dan to regulate his emotional sensitivity. Not only did Dan lack social skills to conduct mature relationships with peers, he was always afraid of doing the wrong thing, being a target of peers' laughter, and being unappreciated by others. Accordingly, Dan needed help to regulate his affective and interpersonal sensitivity.

Dan also needs to learn to regulate sensitivity to internal stimuli. Psychosomatic clients often suffer a difficulty in fine tuning their sensitivity, experiencing both oversensitivity and undersensitivity. Dan exhibited an overawareness to his internal physical cues, sensing the slightest change or tension in his muscles or other body parts, and interpreting this as a signal for distress. He could not differentiate internal cues of tiredness or stiffness from those of pain or illness. Each unpleasant signal was interpreted as sickness. I wanted to decrease his sensitivity to external stressful events, which manifested itself in distressing physical response. I planned to teach him discriminatory practices, whereby he could learn to ignore some sensations, identify other sensations as neutral, and increase his sensitivity to positive sensations.

In terms of developmental tasks affecting my decision about Dan's treatment goals, at age 11, Dan was in middle childhood. His main age-related task was to establish his own identity as a healthy, competitive, capable young child. Assessing Dan's needs in light of developmental roles pinpointed the importance of helping Dan learn to accept himself as a coping person. Continued pain and distress might damage his self-esteem and self-acceptance as a young adolescent.

Although I noticed some problems relating to his acceptance of the family and himself as a member of an immigrant family, therapy did not target this. I felt that the family was not interested in addressing these issues in therapy at that time, and I offered them the option of returning to therapy in the future, if they felt ready to deal with these goals.

Phase 3 of Decision Making: Selecting Who Should Be Treated

As mentioned before, the first intake session was conducted with Dan and his parents together. At that time, I could not pinpoint any specific problems relating directly to Dan's parents. Naturally, parents inevitably comprise an integral part of children's treatment, but I could not identify any particular problematic area of their functioning as parents that would necessitate a focus on the parents' treatment (which later proved wrong). Using Phase 3 to decide on the treatment setting based on developmental considerations (Table 4.4) and the referral type (Table 4.5), I resolved to treat Dan individually. This decision derived from four main considerations: the nature of his psychosomatic complaints, which necessitated individual training in overcoming and accepting methods; the fact that I did not see any reason to treat the parents; Dan's wishes to be treated individually; and Dan's age and cognitive stage, which enabled individual therapy. However, due to the parents' serious concerns about their son, I invited them to join the last 10 minutes of each therapy session. At this stage, assessment had indicated the need to treat Dan individually and the importance of helping him increase social skills, remove anxiety disorder, and regulate his sensitivity. Now I was faced with the next decision: how to treat Dan.

Phase 4 of Decision Making: Selecting Dan's Optimal Treatment Modes

The fourth phase of decision making related to the need to choose techniques for change based on Dan's developmental stage (Table 4.6) and type of referral (Table 4.7). Dan's age and cognitive capability pointed to his ability to enjoy verbal therapy. On the other hand, pain and somatoform disorders can best be treated using nonverbal therapy such as metaphors, imagery, and relaxation. I decided to combine two methods. Verbal cognitive therapy would teach Dan various means to change his way of thinking and to learn self-talk that could improve his coping. As part of those skills, he would need to learn to observe, chart, assess, and evaluate his own behaviors and emotions. Constructivist nonverbal therapy would enable him learn to identify his internal sensations, accepting them and eliminating them, if needed. I decided to help Dan overcome his pain first, and then to try to learn about the source of his stomachaches and how to prevent future pain and improve his quality of life. At this point, we were ready to begin therapy.

Initial Treatment Sessions

As agreed, I started treating Dan individually. The only requests I made of Dan's parents at that point were, first, to refrain from talking with Dan about his pain, referring him to me to discuss that subject, if necessary, and, second, to cease enabling him to stay at home because of pain. These initial requests aimed to eliminate some of the secondary gains Dan received from his symptoms.

My treatment contract with Dan consisted of an agreement that we would start treating him in order to help him cope with the pain, and if we succeeded, he agreed to believe that it was not organic pain and then he would cooperate in trying to change other problematic areas in his functioning.

Only a month later, I had already discovered that not treating the parents was a mistake. The father, upon bringing Dan to a treatment session, suddenly disclosed what he had earlier denied, that he himself had suffered from a stress disorder in the past. It emerged that, by reading behavior and cognitive literature, the father had successfully taught himself relaxation and self-talk. His own success led him to seek out a cognitive therapist to help his son, which led them to me. In another session, when the mother joined us for the last 10 minutes of a session, I observed in the mother a pattern of hysterical responses to various events that resembled Dan's overreactions and the father's prior disorder. I then invited both parents to another session without Dan and asked them about their behavior. They admitted having some marital problems and disclosed that they tended not to express emotions in front of each other, in order to avoid criticism. Each session another parent brought Dan in. At the end of the session they would enter and talk with me for a few minutes. When each of them was with me alone, they would talk about things they did not talk about when they were together. Yet, they were not interested in marital counseling and did not want to address those problems. For example, in the third session, Dan started complaining of a severe headache, looked pale, and cried out: "I'm going to die. I can't stand it." The mother immediately responded by shouting: "Oh, please, God, don't die. This is awful! We need to call a physician! What should I do?" I then turned to Dan and asked him: "Do you think you can go to the bathroom, wash your face, drink some water, and come back?" Dan agreed and after several minutes he returned smiling and said: "Well, I guess it still hurts but it's better." I asked him if he really was going to die, and he replied: "Well, of course not. That's only a way of talking. I'm sick of being in pain." I then asked the mother if she thought her response corresponded with her son's feelings, and she said: "How could I have known it wasn't so bad? He scared me." Dan then said, "You see, she's always so hysterical. That's why I don't want her to be around my friends. I'm ashamed of her." This situation enabled me to understand the family process through which Dan's anxiety level and pains increased. Dan suffered and used extreme terms. His mother was also frightened and used extreme, hysterical responses. Her reactions served both as a reward to him (the family's attention, the mother's concern) and as an extreme model for imitation. By thinking in extreme terms, he did not even try to overcome or resolve the problem of coping with his pain.

After that, I realized that my original decision to treat Dan individually was erroneous and that I would need to treat his parents as well. I then decided to add family meetings to Dan's treatment plan. We continued therapy by treating Dan individually once a week, and treating the whole family once every two weeks. The focus of the family meetings were on working toward learning to react more appropriately to one another, to avoid exaggerated, hysterical responses, and to change the family's communication style.

It was clear to me that Dan was really suffering from physical pain. It is hard to say what caused the pain. I believe it was a combination of several factors: his heightened level of sensitivity in general, his difficulties in coping with stressful emotions, his family's intense sensitivity to his suffering and their efforts to overprotect him, and his insecure feelings with friends on the one hand, and his strong desire to improve his social position and confidence among peers on the other hand. Therefore, I formulated four main aims for Dan's intervention: First, Dan must learn to differentiate the feeling of pain from the thought of impending catastrophe. Second, he must learn to cope with the pain and to decrease it. Third, the family must desist from maintaining his pain or avoidance disorders by reinforcing them. Fourth, Dan must be taught how to deal with his social situation and to develop social skills.

Treating Dan's Pain

The kind of anxieties and somatic symptoms that Dan evidenced suggested the need to use experiential techniques and acceptance methods. Yet, Dan tended to interpret everything as a catastrophe, viewing each internal sensation indiscriminately as a sign of dangerous illness. It was important to help Dan comprehend how his automatic thoughts elicited his stress and fears and thereby exacerbated his pain. A crucial goal was also to help Dan cope with the pain in order to return to school as soon as possible. I therefore decided to use the SCIM model that I described in Chapter 5. However, instead of working, as I am accustomed, on each module as a precursor of the next, in Dan's case I worked simultaneously on all four of the modules together, addressing any or all of them in each session. This approach to the SCIM stemmed from my judgment that the second two self-control modules seemed to be more crucial in Dan's case (increasing awareness to internal stimuli and practicing self-control). Nevertheless, I realized I could not avoid relating to the first two modules (redefinition and linking cause to effect), if I wanted Dan to learn to interpret his sensations differently. I wish to emphasize that, for the purpose of clarity, I will next describe each module separately, in turn, despite the fact that the timing of the modules' utilization in Dan's therapy depended on his feelings or needs that day.

SCIM module 1: Cognitive restructuring, reframing, and redefinition. Dan viewed his pain as an indication of some terrible disease or even as a portent of death. Redefining Dan's pain encompassed several issues such as measuring the pain and giving it a new meaning. First, we redefined sensations and emotions as located on a whole spectrum, rather than as "all or nothing." The "all or nothing" belief incessantly confronted Dan with catastrophe. He had to learn to identify strong pain, mild pain, and very slight pain, and to discriminate between them along a continuum. Second, his pain needed to be redefined as something that caused distress and interfered with his enjoyment from life, rather than as an omen for a terrible future or death. It was very difficult to persuade Dan that the pain was not a sign of something else, but rather constituted the problem itself. I gave him psychological reports to read about pain. I sent him to the library to find and read materials on pain. Yet, mainly, we tried to remember previous incidents of great pain that then disappeared without any disastrous consequences, but which did have other personal or social outcomes. It took several weeks before Dan was able to say: "I hate this pain. It keeps me from going out with my friends" instead of saying: "I'm in pain. I'm sure I'm going to die soon or be hospitalized because this pain means something terrible is going to happen to me."

As we succeeded in redefining Dan's pain, not as a prediction that his life would end but rather as a distress in the present, the problem did not disappear, but Dan was more relaxed and ready to continue and comply with homework assignments. This module helped Dan establish his self-efficacy and his belief in his own ability to overcome, cope, and live with the disorder.

SCIM module 2: Problem analysis. Much effort was invested in therapy into teaching Dan to identify the links between his thoughts, sensations, emotions, and behaviors. I wanted to use cognitive–constructivist techniques to teach Dan about cause and effect, and to understand his role in eliciting his distressful response. By charting and recording at home, and by analyzing those records in the session, we were able to learn about how Dan behaved. When he sensed a change in his muscles, stress, or pain, his automatic thoughts led him to translate the situation into: "Oh, here it comes again. I'm going to be in pain tonight. It'll be terrible. I won't be able to study for the test I have tomorrow." As Dan was saying that to himself, his fear of the distress caused him to look for signals of progressing pain. At the same time, he would contract his muscles. This would cause the pain to be stronger. The fear and anxiety would facilitate the sense of pain, and Dan would become hysterical.

After Dan learned to identify the link between his thoughts, emotions, and behaviors, he was trained in trying to disconnect this link. First, the use of self-talk was introduced to prevent situations where the slightest awareness of pain produced great distress. He was taught to practice saying to himself: "It's normal to feel what I feel. Everyone has similar sensations. It's not a sign of anything. Only dead people don't feel anything. I'm happy I can feel." He was also trained to look for good sensations, and to allow himself to feel satisfied that he was able to identify a sense of being relaxed and happy, but this will be described later on. Dan was given the assignment of talking to himself every day whenever he felt pain or anticipated feeling pain. Initially, he used written notes that we prepared in the session, because it was very difficult for him to think of something positive when he felt pain. Later on, as he progressed, he was able to make statements up on his own and no longer needed the preprepared notes.

Then, Dan learned to try changing his anxiety-evoking sensation via imagery exercises and relaxation exercises. Last, he learned to pursue enjoyable activities that he could initiate instead of thinking about his terrible condition.

SCIM module 3: Attentional focus. At this stage, we focused mainly on constructivist techniques, and I believe that this module offered the main techniques for working with Dan. As mentioned before, I wanted to desensitize Dan's attention to his negative internal stimuli while, at the same time, increasing his awareness to positive sensations.

While trying to decide on a strategy to help him, I thought I should, first of all, help Dan meet his pain, embrace it, and accept it. I expected this approach would mobilize his motivation to work toward improving his coping in general. At the same time, I hoped to learn more about Dan's problem, contributing to a more effective design of the intervention for change.

From the way Dan coped with his pain, I realized he was trying to avoid it and overcome it, not live with it or accept it. I explained to him the rationale for our treatment:

> Often, when people try to run away from fears or pain, they find those emotions running after them. The faster they run, the more they fear the pain or fears will catch them. However, when we stand up and embrace the unpleasant emotions (fear, anxiety, pain, stress), they become smaller and smaller. And then, from very close up, we can see that they are not so problematic

after all, and we can actually deal with them. Therefore, the very first thing we are going to learn is to stop running away and, instead, to get acquainted with the pain.

Dan, who had a great sense of humor and no problems in expressing his thoughts, answered immediately: "Are you sure you are a licensed therapist? Because I've met three like you before [in school and at the hospital], and all of them tried to teach me how to overcome it, but you're asking me to do the opposite. If my situation gets worse, my parents will sue you ..." Nevertheless, Dan was very cooperative as we started.

Using mirror time (Mahoney, 1991) I asked Dan to get acquainted with his pain. He had to look at himself in the mirror while in pain; charting exercises that helped him understand the outcomes of his behavior before, during, and after pain; imagery exercises to facilitate his meeting up with his pain; mindfulness exercises; and a focus on openness to experiences. Csikszentmihalyi (1966) proposed that the best way to gain control over something is to open oneself up to experience and temporarily let go of control. This was the purpose of the intervention's emphasis on getting acquainted with the pain.

The first part of getting acquainted with the pain was for Dan to see what he looked like while suffering pain. Mahoney (1991) suggested this technique to help people meet themselves. Many clients use the mirror as a medium for initiating or continuing dialogues, especially when they are accustomed to hiding beyond intellectual exchanges. Some individuals experience strong reactions to eye contact, and the strategy of asking clients to open and close their eyes can elicit significant responses. Some clients also find it helpful to listen to guiding questions.

Dan was instructed to sit in front of a mirror during our session, getting to know his facial expressions while I had to guess, according to those facial expressions, how strong his pains were. Soon, we concluded that he responded indiscriminately to each pain as if he was in the worst possible agony. From the way he looked, talked, or acted, no one could differentiate between severe pains and mild aches. He was asked to prepare a ladder of facial expressions. The ladder included several emotions, such as happy and relaxed ("My eyes are shining, I'm laughing, and no muscles are showing in my face") and also feeling severe pain ("My eyes are almost closed, my mouth looks funny, and I can see some strange lines or is it muscles in my face?"). In rating his feelings by giving them numbers, Dan said that 10 was the best feeling and 0 was the worst. His homework for the coming week was to stand twice daily in front of the mirror, once while feeling good and once while suffering, and to record the characteristics and peculiarities of his facial expressions at those times.

The second part of getting acquainted with pain consisted of studying its outcomes: how he behaved afterwards, how it affected his relationships with parents and friends, how he functioned differently when relaxed and when suffering. After this session, Dan was assigned as homework the task of recording his behaviors and thoughts every day, and trying to pinpoint all the advantages and disadvantages of being in pain. Without being asked, he also noted his maternal grandmother's facial expression while he was in pain. I already knew from the intake session that the grandmother was living with them, but I was not aware before then of her role in reinforcing Dan's problem. The grandmother and Dan were very close, and she was very overprotective. He laughed while saying: "You can look at grandma and know that I'm in pain." I asked his grandmother to join the next family session, at which time I assigned both his grandmother and parents the task of trying to confuse Dan by purposely changing their facial expressions. I also asked Dan to attempt to confuse his family by not letting them know what he was really feeling. They really enjoyed that session, which was peppered with many jokes and laughs, but it also tangibly increased the family's understanding of my intention when I asked for their cooperation in stopping their secondary reinforcement and maintenance of Dan's pain.

The third part of getting acquainted with the pain incorporated attempts to learn what the pain looked like and to try to change it, mainly via mindfulness exercises. The practice of mindfulness exercises invites clients to attend to themselves, to let themselves focus on the body, just like in meditation, when one can ignore internal interference and can concentrate, without thinking about what is occurring in one's inside (Mahoney, 1991).

Another technique we used was imagery training. At first, we searched for the pain. I asked Dan to imagine himself as a very small figure the size of a match, and to enter into himself for a trip inside his body. I asked him to walk around and see what he saw and felt from inside. Through the proper use of mental imagery, one can achieve an immediate sense of self-confidence, develop more energy and stamina, and tap one's own mind for numerous productive purposes. Associative imagery can be most useful in tracking down reasons behind everyday upsets (Lazarus, 1984).

During these internal excursions, Dan expressed discomfort in two places inside his body. As we reached his throat, he said it was too hot, too crowded, and he felt he was going to vomit. In addition, as we neared his stomach, Dan pronounced: "Oh, here is a whole big mess. I can't see my way through. It's too dark. I hate to be here, I want out." He insisted on ending the exercise then and there. To improve his feeling, I redefined his demand to stop the exercise as: "Hey, that's wonderful. I see you don't like your pain. That's the first sign that we'll be able to get rid of it. Could you imagine what would happen if you said you loved being in there and that it was great in there?"

After he relaxed, I asked his permission to get closer to the pain once more, and, after a little hesitation, he agreed. So, we practiced another exercise, this time a metaphoric one that we recorded on audiotape. I asked him to close his eyes, take a deep breath, release all the tension, and feel his body parts becoming heavy. Then I asked him to try and see if he could notice the pain. Dan pointed towards his stomach and mentioned that on that day he was in great pain and did not even go to school. I asked him to see if he could locate the pain – its exact place and shape. He described it as a small concentrated ball. I asked about movement, and Dan said it could not move. It was too heavy. I asked him to try and very slowly move it around. At first, this was difficult for him to do, but after a few minutes he reported that it was moving very slowly. I asked about its color, and Dan replied that it was deep purple. When he added that he hated purple and liked green, I asked if he could imagine rivers of green streaming from his brain to color his purple ball. Slowly, he could see it becoming green, and then we started working to move the ball toward the direction of his hand. At the end, I asked Dan to push it into his fist and hold it there tightly so that it would not disappear. This imagery exercise lasted the whole session. At the end, Dan announced that he did not feel any pain other than the muscles in his fists. I asked him to rate his pain on a scale of 0 to 10 in whichever direction he chose. He said that 0 indicated a terrible feeling and that before we started it was at 0, but now it was at about 8, which was quite all right. I asked Dan to practice listening to the audiotaped exercise daily in order to practice learning about his pain: how big it was, where it was located, its shape and colors, etc.

Later that day, Dan called me by phone, crying that his pain had returned 5 hours later. I instructed him to continue listening to the tape. At home, he did not succeed in decreasing the pain, and he could not reach a comfort rate of more than 5. However, after 3 weeks of practice, he was able to raise this to 6 or 7, and only once did his pain return to 0. With that level of feeling, Dan was able to go to school and function. He insisted that the pain was still hiding somewhere. We made a deal that he was not allowed to stay at home unless he felt wonderful and decided to have a fun time with his parents once in a while.

At this time, Dan' s parents were urgently invited to school one day because (as the teacher said) "Dan was in terrible condition, he was suffering a lot, and should be taken home immediately." I then decided to go to the school. I met with the teacher and school counselor. I realized they were reinforcing his behavior and contributing to the sense of panic the mother felt. I advised them to ignore his complaints, to refrain from calling the parents, and if he persisted in feeling bad, to send him to drink water or wash his face. I also asked them not to release him from school assignments and to make it clear to him that, if he skipped school, he would have to complete all the missing assignments.

SCIM module 4: Self-control exercises. The last module, practicing self-control skills, actually comprised the application of all the skills learned in the other modules. Dan practiced self-talk, self-recording, and self-evaluation. He assessed his progress, checked all his records, and realized that over the last few weeks he had attended school every day, even on the first day of the week, the most difficult day for him after being home for the weekend. Also, he realized that he still suffered from headaches and stomachaches but that these were not very painful, and they did not prevent him from functioning. He was very happy to admit that: "I believe I'm managing pretty well, and I've been able to overcome most of my problems."

As Dan progressed, he was guided in an imagery exercise where he had to imagine himself without pain. He practiced this exercise within sessions and as homework. We called this exercise: "My fantasyland." At first, Dan said it was impossible to see himself without pain. I asked him when he thought it could be possible – in a year? 3 years? 10 years? 20? Then I asked him to fly off into the future, as far as necessary in order to view himself without pain. The instructions were: "Now you're flying to the land of your desire. This land can be a real place you've visited before and wish to return to; it can be a place you've never been but heard of; or it can be a place you invent, your fantasyland. In this land, you feel all the feelings you want to, you sense all the senses that are important to you. You are healthy, happy, relaxed, and enjoying yourself. Notice all the noises around you, look at the colors, pay attention to the climate and the land, and then look at yourself and note the way you look while you're experiencing all those emotions, sensations, and feelings."

Slowly, Dan was able to view himself without pain. He could also chart longer and longer periods of time without pain, and his pain ratings decreased to 2 or 3 (on the aforementioned scale of 10 as the worst pain and 0 as not suffering at all). His comfort scale was in the opposite direction, with 10 symbolizing the best feeling and 0 the worst.

The stage of therapeutic work on getting acquainted with the pain took us about 6 weeks. As he progressed, more and more of the work was assigned as homework, freeing time within the sessions for other kinds of interventions.

Treating Dan's Social Problems

As described above, Dan seemed very anxious about his social position, his peer relationships, and his capacity to handle difficult social situations. He worried about acting foolishly, being laughed at, or being different from others. Hence, Dan needed help reducing his anxiety through social skills training. In addition, Dan had undergone some aversive, violent peer interactions, and he lacked the necessary social skills to conduct mature relationships with peers, which would increase his self-confidence and self-esteem. Dan needed assertiveness training, that is, teaching him how to appropriately fight back or stand up for his rights.

Moreover, it came to my attention that the heterogeneous demographic makeup of the school population also comprised a social challenge for Dan. He needed to be taught to develop and increase his social skills mainly toward the direction of choosing friends who were more like him, with whom he could find mutual interests. Although the students in his school from the north of the city were generally from a highly educated, high social class background like himself,

Dan was attracted to those students from the south who were from a low social class background with a high rate of parental unemployment and who were more aggressive both verbally and physically. Dan wanted to join the children from the other part of the city, who made fun of the diligent students, did not do their homework, and were busy having a good time, laughing at and teasing others, and hitting each other. Dan, who was talented, clever, and even looked different from this peer group, was not accepted by them despite his attempts to join in.

For the next three months, we discussed topics such as how one chooses friends and what makes friends really feel like friends. We talked about his expectations and future aims, trying to pinpoint what made him happy. He chose some after school activities that seemed appealing, joining a basketball team and a youth group. He made a list of friends in school, trying to estimate who could be good, true friends. We practiced methods of picking friends, using role-playing to simulate social conversations. In addition, we used methods of self-evaluation and self-complimenting to increase his self-acceptance and self-assurance.

Dan started going out and taking part in class activities. He would join peers' games during school recesses, and he often met with two or three good friends over the weekend and went with them to see a movie. He did not like crowded parties or "hanging out" with the whole class in the streets, but, from time to time, he participated in these activities too.

Phase 5 of Decision Making: Evaluating Dan at the End of Therapy and Maintaining Treatment Outcomes

Evaluation. Dan's baseline assessment had pinpointed three main issues: his psychosomatic complaints, his avoidance of school, and his lack of healthy social relationships. This information had been given by the parents, by Dan, and from observing Dan's behavior and pain.

According to the guidelines I outlined in Table 4.8, the selection of evaluation methods should consider the treatment goals. Thus, the appropriate evaluation tools for Dan, whose goals were to increase social behavior and remove anxiety, included Dan's own reports on his emotional and social functioning, and parental reports as well. To evaluate Dan's progress, then, I conducted a session with him and his parents, asking for their feedback. Both of the parents and Dan reported dramatic change in all three issues. Also, in my observations of Dan over the last few weeks, I had not seen him in pain.

The first part of the treatment (decreasing the pain) very dramatically presented rapid outcomes. The acute pain decreased after the first 6 weeks. Dan continued to suffer occasional pain for the next 5 months, until it disappeared completely. The second part (imparting social skills) was slower, characterized by small changes that took longer to achieve.

The biweekly family meetings helped change the family's communication style, imparting the family members with more appropriate skills for communicating with one another. For example, the mother learned to react more calmly to Dan and to refrain from panicking. Dan decreased his level of ironic and cynical communication with his parents. Also, it seemed as if the family members were better able to conduct real conversation, rather than settling only for jokes or sarcasm.

Maintenance. At this point, I instigated the transition to the maintenance stage of intervention. Dan was very pleased to receive my affirmation that he no longer needed intense therapy. We agreed that Dan would call me once in two to three weeks for a follow-up session. I still wanted him to keep records of his behaviors and sensations. Dan called me twice to tell me how happy he was, and how well he progressed, and asked to stop recording and charting. I was convinced that his new social relationships would be a natural reinforcement for him, and agreed to his requests.

I saw Dan again one year after termination of therapy. Now age 13, he came to consult me as to whether he could join a citywide swim team without fear of harming himself. Although his apprehension about his body continued to a minor degree, Dan did not report any pain. His complaints typified those of children his age: too many hours in school, too much homework, overly strict parents who did not allow him to stay out all night. He also reported that he was satisfied with his social relations.

Two years later I saw him once more. He came to consult with me about his girlfriend. He was unsure as to whether or not he should talk with her about something that bothered him, and he wanted to hear my opinion. He sounded like any other normal adolescent occupied with first intimacy and love relationships.

10

Enuresis

LITERATURE REVIEW

Children's bedwetting is a socially significant problem, and professional consensus about its treatment is still lacking (Houts et al., 1994; Rappaport, 1993). Enuresis is considered to be one of the most common behavior problems among children (Rutter et al., 1973). Enuresis is defined as a repeated voiding of urine into the bed or clothes. The behavior is clinically significant as manifested by either a frequency of twice a week for at least three consecutive months or the presence of clinically significant distress or impairment in social, academic, or other important areas of functioning. The chronological age for diagnosis is at least 5 years. Also, the behavior is not due exclusively to the direct physiological effect of a substance or a general medical condition (*DSM-IV*; American Psychiatric Association, 1994). The frequency of enuretic children in the population reaches as high as 30% at the age of 5 and drops in prevalence with increased age (Doleys, 1977), demonstrating a higher frequency among boys than girls (De Jong, 1973; Doleys, 1977). The high predominance of nocturnal enuresis during childhood and even adolescence has been widely documented in the literature (Azrin & Thiens, 1978; Doleys, 1977; Fielding & Doleys, 1988; Houts et al., 1994).

Enuretic children comprise a heterogeneous group with different etiologies and behavioral problems (Fielding & Doleys, 1988). Most enuretic children exhibit nocturnal (nighttime) enuresis. Some present diurnal (daytime) enuresis, and the minority present both nocturnal and diurnal enuresis. Among enuretic children, the majority evidence primary enuresis (i.e. continuous bedwetting since birth, defined as a child who has never had six continuous months of being dry). Those who exhibit secondary enuresis (i.e. bedwetting that occurs after at least a six-month continuous period of dryness; Houts et al., 1994), usually present a regression in the normal developmental toilet training response.

Most enuretic children have a clear familial history, that is, where at least one parent was enuretic as a child. However, some children show no association to family history. In a study carried out in Spain among 70 enuretic children aged 5–14-years-old, 69% had a family history of enuresis, and 54% had first-degree relatives (mainly siblings) who had enuresis (Rey-Sanchez et al., 1995). Enuretic children may or may not demonstrate accompanying behavioral problems (Ronen & Wozner, 1995). Rey-Sanchez et al. found that 60% of their sample did not present other psychopathology. The remaining children were diagnosed with encopresis and developmental disorders. Most children with enuresis reveal no clear association to major behavior problems other than those directly associated with enuresis, such as immature behavior, low self-esteem, and poor self-image (De Jong, 1973; Doleys, 1977; Rutter et al., 1973).

Enuresis affects children's functioning in different ways in their personal, familial, academic, and social relations. In the personal realm, enuretic children are characterized by low self-confidence, low self-esteem, and feelings of helplessness and distress. The familial functioning is affected because enuresis often becomes the center of the family and the cause of arguments, punishments, and parental and sibling resentment. In the academic realm, children often give up trying to cope with academic tasks, rationalizing that if they cannot control a simple thing such as the bladder, how can they cope with complicated learning processes? Social relations are affected because the children are afraid that the terrible secret will be discovered; therefore, they avoid going on trips, to camps, sleeping out overnight, or asking friends over (Houts et al., 1994).

Over the years, enuresis has been attributed with different causes and explanations. Those interested in medical and physical etiology have underscored EEG patterns, lack of ADH hormones, sleeping patterns, and other factors, but the bladder itself has received the most attention. In order to stay dry, one must learn both to develop and to control strong bladder muscles. Research concerning the bladder has emphasized the fact that the problem is not whether the bladder is sufficiently strong or large, but whether the child can withstand the unpleasant stimuli and continue restraining (Fielding & Doleys, 1988). Genetic explanations relate enuresis to the high parent–child enuresis association, whereby most enuretic children have at least one parent who was enuretic as a child (Bakwin, 1971).

Behavioral and familial components of enuresis have been attributed with playing a central role, where enuresis is conceptualized either as a behavior that children learn by modeling and reinforcement, or as a skills deficit necessitating training (Azrin & Foxx, 1974; Azrin et al., 1974). The cognitive component of enuresis relates to the child's cognitive skills, which maintain the problem and avoid its solution. Misconceptions such as: "It is a sickness, and I cannot solve it" or "Why should I try to cope with something that does not depend on me?" could hinder a solution to the problem. More recently, enuresis has been conceived as a biobehavioral problem (Houts, 1991), that is, a physical problem with behavioral and psychological causes and consequences (Jones, 1960).

Treatment

Various methods have been developed for the treatment of enuresis. Research reports present a high rate of success (between 70% and 90%) immediately following therapy. Most of these studies refer only to those children who remained in therapy. These studies ignore the high percentage of dropouts (about 30%), and the subsequent relapse rate (as high as 50%) in the three to six months after termination of therapy (Azrin & Foxx, 1974; Doleys, 1977; Fielding & Doleys, 1988; Ronen et al., 1992; Taylor & Turner, 1975).

The most common treatments for enuresis are pharmacological, family, behavioral, and cognitive methods.

Pharmacology targets the biological and genetic problems (Houts, 1991) by prescription of medications, especially Minerine, Imipramine, and other tricyclic antidepressants (Blackwell & Currah, 1973; Johnson, 1980).

Various kinds of family therapies have been applied to enuresis. Bellver-Cebria (1999) reported a successful treatment of an 8-year-old child. The treatment focused on improving family dynamics, changing parent–child interactions, and reducing maladaptive behavior. Other modes of family therapy and family counseling are based on behavioral therapy. Such treatments are often directed toward instructing parents to change their responses to the child's bedwetting (Morgan & Young, 1975). Parents are trained in procedures for a full cleaning practice, based on rearranging environmental conditions to facilitate the child's acquisition of appropriate control responses (Azrin & Foxx, 1974; Azrin et al., 1974).

Behavioral and cognitive techniques have been developed to target the elimination of primary nocturnal enuresis by treating the children themselves. Retention control training focuses on the bladder, emphasizing the limited functional capacity of enuretic children, and suggesting exercises that foster awareness of bladder sensations and increase bladder capacity (Doleys et al., 1977; Fielding, 1980; Fielding & Doleys, 1988; Ronen & Abraham, 1995). Other child-centered techniques aim to change the outcome of the urination problem either by reinforcing dryness through a token economy program (Finley et al., 1973) or by punishing enuresis and reinforcing dryness. The most popular technique for elimination of enuresis is the bell-and-pad method (Berg et al., 1982; Mowrer & Mowrer, 1938). This technique uses an alarm that rings each time the child begins to wet the bed. The technique helps in the elimination of enuresis in two ways. One, the sound of the alarm at night and the need to wake up, go to the toilet to continue emptying oneself, and to change the bedding, all serve as a punishment that teaches the child to avoid enuresis. Two, the alarm serves as a cue that teaches the child to identify the internal stimuli of a full bladder.

Several controlled studies and meta-analyses during the last few years have investigated the efficacy of different techniques for the elimination of enuresis. Alcazar et al. (1999) conducted a meta-analysis of 14 independent studies conducted in Spain. They compared the effectiveness of three main behavioral interventions: bell-and-pad (alarm), retention control training, and dry bed training. Significant differences were found among the three techniques, and the dry bed training and bell-and-pad technique were shown to be most effective for eliminating enuresis.

Almost every method that has been applied to enuresis control has described the need to impart the child with self-control skills. Such skills can help the child to postpone the need to urinate, to wake up at night, or to invest effort into solving the problem (i.e. to gain motivation for avoiding drinking at night, going to sleep early, and taking responsibility for remaking the wet bed) (Azrin & Foxx, 1974). Nevertheless, none of the aforementioned methods views enuresis as deriving from deficiencies in self-control and therefore as being capable of elimination through imparting self-control skills.

Ronen and colleagues (1992) suggested that self-control skill deficits might provide an explanation for the gender and familial characteristics of enuresis. The gender differences in enuretic children resemble the differential self-control levels found among boys and girls in self-control studies that measure skills such as the ability to overcome temptation, delay gratification, and overcome pain, pressure, or disturbing feelings (Kendall & Wilcox, 1980). Boys' higher frequency of enuresis may be related to their lower self-control skills. Research on self-control skills in adults also demonstrates higher self-control levels in women as compared to men. The familial association found between enuretic children and their parents (Bakwin, 1971; Fielding & Doleys, 1988) can also be compared to correlations found between parents' self-control and children's self-control (Ronen et al., 1992).

Eliminating enuresis can thus be directly linked to cognitive skills of self-control such as self-efficacy (Bandura, 1969), one's belief system, and expectations (Beck et al., 1979; Ellis, 1962). These skills facilitate the child's attempts to overcome pressure, disturbing behavior, pain, and stress and to postpone gratification (Copeland, 1982; Thorsen & Mahoney, 1974).

Ronen and her colleagues (Ronen et al., 1992, 1995; Ronen & Wozner, 1995) proposed a cognitive model that focuses on the acquisition of self-control skills rather than on conditioning. The approach uses corrective methods such as self-talk, self-monitoring, self-evaluation, and self-reinforcement. Once acquired, these self-control skills may be expected to remain available for a prolonged period and are not subject to the same extinction processes as are conditioned responses.

The proposed self-control training for enuresis emphasizes a link between the physical, behavioral, familial, and cognitive elements of enuresis. The role of self-control skills is accentuated, not only for developing but also for maintaining appropriate toilet habits, suggesting these skills' importance in facilitating treatment outcomes. The acquisition of self-control skills enables the child to identify his or her automatic, habitual way of thinking and change it into a mediated, planned way of thinking. It facilitates the child's recognition of the role of thought in emotional arousal, allowing the child to overcome disturbing emotions, to learn the cause for his or her behavior, and to acquire effective techniques for behavior change (Copeland, 1982; Kendall & Braswell, 1985; Meichenbaum, 1979, 1985).

The following case study illustrates the application of my SCIM training model (described in Chapter 5) to a preadolescent enuretic girl.

THE CASE OF SHARON'S BEDWETTING

At the time of her referral, 12-year-old Sharon was suffering from primary nocturnal enuresis. As Sharon and her parents arrived at the clinic for the first intake session, her mother said: "Now you see why we have only one child. Since Sharon never stopped wetting the bed, I couldn't stand the idea of having more bedwetters at home. Could you take her, and send her back to me when she is dry?" This introduction made me feel that there were probably a handful of familial and parenting problems connected to the etiology of Sharon's enuresis, and I decided that a focus on assessing the parents and family was in order.

Assessing Sharon and Her Family

As mentioned in Chapter 4, we begin our assessment as soon as the client enters the clinic and we see the client and the family for the first time. The presented problem was enuresis. Enuresis, as a problem that occurs at home, is only known to the child and her family (excluding the need for teacher reports, as recommended in Table 4.2 for referrals with the goal of decreasing behaviors such as bedwetting). I determined, therefore, that Sharon's assessment should relate to two main issues. The first concerned the specific nature of her enuresis, which could best be identified using parents' and children's interviews and by charting Sharon's enuresis pattern every day. The second involved family relationships and the family's way of relating to the problem, which could be gleaned via family interviewing. This selection of self-reports and parents' reports as the assessment methods of choice is advocated for adolescents aged 12–18 (see Table 4.3).

To learn more about the family, I asked Sharon to demonstrate their relationships to me by making a live sculpture of the family. Sharon moved both her parents into a position of hugging each other and then put herself in the middle between them. When I asked her how she felt inside, she answered, "warm and protected." I asked everyone to decide if they felt comfortable in this position, or if they wished to change anything. The only thing the father said was to the mother: "I love you to hug me but, please, let go a little bit so I'll be able to look around...!"

I then asked Sharon to draw her family as animals. She drew a picture of her mother as a dog and explained: "She barks to intimidate but she never bites, just like that saying of 'barking dogs don't bite!' She's also very loyal to the family and she protects us all." Sharon drew her father as a bird and said, "Birds always fly away to look for food but they come back to the nest to feed the little birds and they are good parents, but they need their freedom and can't manage well in a cage." She drew herself as a cat because: "Cats are proud, spoiled, and loved."

In another session, I met Sharon's parents alone, asking them about the sculpture and the father's need to breathe, as well as about Sharon's drawing of her father as a bird with the focus on the father's need for freedom. They laughed and said that they had both grown up as only children in overprotecting homes. Both of them described how they cared very much for the family, had good caring relationships between themselves, and felt they loved each other. They had decided not to have more than one child, just to make sure that they could give this child everything she needed without having to divide their attention. The mother added that she had never worked out of the house, and she was very dependent on the father, who needed his freedom, however. They said it was a family joke to talk about the father's freedom, but that, actually, the father was even more involved in and concerned about everything than the mother was.

Sharon's mother, despite her caring attitude, was highly frustrated by the fact that she could not help Sharon stop wetting the bed. The mother constantly shifted from supporting and helping, to being angry and punishing, to trying to be indifferent. She worried a great deal about how Sharon would manage to live with the enuresis and what kind of damage it would cause in her future. The father, on the other hand, said he was also an enuretic child, and he was sure Sharon would overcome it in the future and that there was nothing to worry about.

In the intake session, they told me that Sharon had already tried everything. She had been in play therapy for two years at the age of 6, used the bell-and-pad method at the age of 10, and immediately afterwards had taken medications (minerine). Nothing had helped. In the past, she used to wet the bed 2 to 3 times every night, but at the time of referral she was wetting the bed five to six nights a week, only once a night. She was a good student and had many friends; however, she was afraid of inviting friends over because she feared they would notice the wet laundry. She never slept out of the house nor did she go on school trips or to camp because of her problem.

Phase 1 of Decision Making: Does Sharon Need Therapy or Not?

The decision as to whether or not Sharon needed treatment was a function of the four variables presented in Chapter 4 (see Table 4.1). Sharon's presenting problem met the *DSM-IV* criteria for enuresis (American Psychiatric Association, 1994). At age 12, almost nightly bedwetting pointed to the fact that this problem required treatment. The frequency of her disorder had not improved over the years, so there was no reason to wait for spontaneous recovery.

In terms of developmental variables, enuresis at Sharon's age was deviant by all standards. It was common neither in her age group, nor in her sex group or cultural group. Sharon's behavior was clearly deviant and should have been resolved long ago.

With regard to the child and family variables, both Sharon and her parents demonstrated high motivation for change. They all suffered from the disorder and wished to resolve it. Being enuretic affected Sharon's ability to leave the house and participate in age-appropriate social activities such as sleeping overnight at a friend's, going on a class trip, or attending camp. Sharon avoided these activities for fear that she would wet the bed. She also developed a sense of helplessness and difficulties in gaining self-confidence and positive self-evaluation, due to her failure to control her bladder.

In terms of treatment variables, it has been well documented that enuresis can be resolved through therapy. The rate of success is very high, and chances were good that treating Sharon would eliminate the bedwetting. The longstanding nature of her problem suggested that it would not change without intervention. Sharon's motivation and cooperation in the first intake session highlighted the likelihood that she could develop a good therapeutic relationship, which would be conducive to designing an optimal treatment for resolving the problem and helping her cope better.

My conclusion at this stage was that Sharon clearly needed to be in therapy, and that therapy would very likely eliminate her enuresis.

Phase 2 of Decision Making: Classifying Sharon's Referral and Goals for Change

The second phase of decision making (see Chapter 4) requires the classification of children's referred disorders in light of the goals of intervention and developmental considerations. As seen in Table 4.2, considering the four common reasons for childhood referrals (decreasing behavior, increasing behavior, removing anxiety, and facilitating development), Sharon's enuresis was a disorder requiring elimination (decreasing behavior) due to its overly frequent occurrence. The treatment goals would therefore be to impart Sharon with deficient self-control skills and help her learn to delay temptation and to tolerate frustration.

At the age of early adolescence, youngsters are beginning to become occupied with the need to separate from their parents, develop their own identity, and get involved in social activities (see Table 4.3). Because of her enuresis, Sharon avoided many social activities. Moreover, as an overprotected only child, she found it difficult to separate from her parents and develop autonomous functioning. These problems implied the need to address her place in the family and the family's role in her disorder.

Phase 3 of Decision Making: Selecting Who Should Be Treated

Developmental considerations (see Table 4.4) as well as Sharon's type of referred problem (see Table 4.5) both indicated the need for Sharon to receive individual treatment techniques. Treatment should be directed to impart Sharon with the needed skills to eliminate her enuresis. In addition, family supervision would be necessary. Supervision would involve the parents in promoting Sharon's ability to take on more responsibility, enabling her to separate from her parents and learn to be more independent.

Assessment of Sharon's family had revealed their good relationships, love and affection, and ability to talk about emotions. It seemed that there were no particularly difficult emotions or problems in the family. I believed Sharon's disorder was related to educational problems rather than to psychological pathology. In other words, the parents were very protective, spoiling their daughter, and had difficulty coping with their worries about her and letting her be independent. They also felt helpless coping with the disorder, moving from one extreme response to the other and thereby confusing their daughter.

I could not give a full explanation as to the cause of enuresis, but I could see how the parents were ineffective in handling it. I noted that Sharon was a nice, intelligent girl; yet she had been overly dependent on her parents when it came to her previous attempts to cease her bedwetting. For example, it was the parents who had ensured she took her medication every night, because "she tended to forget." While using the bell-and-pad technique, the parents set up the equipment every night and came to awaken her when the alarm rang, because "she couldn't hear anything while sleeping."

It seemed very clear that Sharon needed to take on more responsibility, and especially to learn to view the enuresis as "her problem" and to deal with its consequences. The parents, on the other hand, needed to learn to give up control and let Sharon take responsibility instead of them.

Phase 4 of Decision Making: Selecting Sharon's Optimal Treatment Modes

Tables 4.6 and 4.7 present the selection of treatment methods in light of developmental criteria and Sharon's specific disorder. Sharon's preadolescent stage allowed for her to participate in verbal therapy. Often at this age, young adolescents even reject nonverbal therapy, thinking it too childish. Sharon had already acquired the necessary cognitive skills to engage in verbal therapy, and this was selected as the treatment of choice. Sharon's problem, enuresis, could also be best treated with verbal methods, due to the need to demonstrate, impart, and practice skills conducive to decreasing her unwanted behaviors and enhancing self-control.

I determined that therapy would include two parts: (a) supervision sessions with the parents, which would be directed toward teaching the parents how to deal with Sharon's bedwetting, how to be insistent and consistent in their demands, and how to reinforce mature instead of immature behavior; and (b) self-control training with Sharon in the presence of her parents. I emphasized treating Sharon in her parents' presence because this was not family therapy. We did not deal with familial issues but, rather, with Sharon's ability for self-control. However, I felt it important in this particular family that the parents be present. I wanted them to see, hear, and be aware of the way I was treating Sharon, both as a model for them in how to talk to and treat her, and as a helping agent to facilitate her practicing and generalizing the skills at home.

Starting Intervention: Family Supervision

As a first step, I asked the parents to start demanding that Sharon take care of the wet laundry, wash it, and make the bed. At first, the mother said "But there's no need, because the machine washes it." However, I insisted on it, and they understood it should be part of the program.

In the family supervision sessions, we practiced techniques and methods in helping the parents demand help, independence, and responsibility from Sharon. At first, Sharon did not like the idea, but soon she understood it was important for her as well, and she was ready to comply with the treatment assignments.

Self-Control Therapy with Sharon

The SCIM model was implemented to offer Sharon the requisite self-control skills for eliminating enuresis, including the four training modules presented in Table 5.1.

SCIM module 1: Cognitive restructuring and redefinition. The first module was directed toward learning to identify Sharon's own meaning making of the enuresis and changing Sharon's conceptions about her inability to be responsible for her behavior. Like other enuretic children, Sharon looked at bedwetting as something beyond her control, something that occurred because "it just escaped" or because she "didn't feel it" or "was sick." As constructivist therapy proposes, clients are responsible for the way they construe and construct their world. Sharon construed her life as an enuretic girl, who could not control her behavior, and it was something that just happened to her. Therefore, I used Socratic questions and paradoxical examples to help her and her parents understand that bedwetting does not depend on bad luck or illness but, rather, is a function of motivation and will power. I attempted first to tackle her conceptions about not feeling anything at night and her belief that this prevented her from controlling her bedwetting:

Therapist: What do you think, why do you wet your bed at night?
Sharon: I don't feel anything when I'm asleep. It's not my fault. It's not up to me.
T: Let's check this out. How many times do you fall out of your bed at night?
S: Never.
T: How come?
S: Because I don't move when I sleep.
T: Really? Let's check it out: Please find a nice position in which you'll feel comfortable. Now, I want you to stay in the same position and not move at all.

We continued talking, and after two minutes Sharon started fidgeting from side to side.

T: You see, Sharon, after two minutes you already moved. Why?
S: It hurts. I can't stay in the same position all day long.
T: You know, the same thing happens at night. You feel uncomfortable, and for that reason you move from one side to the other.
S: Well, then, I guess that when I get close to the edge of the bed I just turn to the other side.
T: Aha! Let's see something else. Did it ever happen during the winter that your blanket fell off?
S: Sure!
T: What did you do?
S: I woke up and covered myself.
T: What happens in the summer when you are very hot at night?
S: I throw the blanket off.
T: You see, even while you are asleep there are things you feel. You feel the edge of the bed, you feel cold, you feel hot. Even when you're asleep, you feel certain things.
S: Right.

At this point, I was interested in attacking another automatic thought that she had, her construction of the event: the belief that bedwetting was out of her control. I asked her to please stand up and hop on one foot. She did so, and I asked her if she could sit down and then get up and do it again. She looked at me, hesitating, and then I asked if she thought it could be possible to be able to know how to hop at 5 p.m. but be unable to do so at 6 p.m.? Or could it be she knew how to do it on Monday but not on Sunday? As she laughed, I told her that the fact she was not wetting herself during the day meant that she knew how to delay the temptation of emptying her bladder and that she could control the muscles of her bladder. The fact that she was able to stay dry about one to two nights a week also meant that there was nothing wrong with her bladder; instead, the problem was probably due to the fact she did not know what she needed to do in order to change her bedwetting. That would be the purpose of our therapy: to learn and practice methods for becoming dry.

As a homework assignment, she was asked to keep a chart on the frequency of wetting as well as to observe her own behavior, noting the position in which she was going to sleep versus the position in which she awakened, and whether she heard or felt anything while sleeping. Also, she was asked to try to pinpoint the time and manner of wetting the bed ("Did you do it all at once, or slowly throughout the whole night?") as well as the time she had her last drink before going to sleep and the time of going to sleep.

In the next session, we started by checking her homework assignment. Sharon had become a real scientist and observed her own behavior. She laughed, telling me that she had discovered that sometimes she woke up on the other end of the bed. She mentioned that twice she woke up during the night and went to the toilet.

SCIM module 2: Problem analysis. After the first four sessions that addressed Sharon's conceptions, automatic thoughts, and misconceptions, we started to target the second training module, which aimed to elucidate the cause–effect link and to focus on rational analysis of the problem. The purpose of these sessions was to teach Sharon about the whole process that culminated in urination. She learned how drinking fills the bladder and causes the unpleasant pressure that is transferred to the brain, and how the brain then "sends" commands to the valve to open and release the urine, an action which ends the unpleasant sensation. It was important for me to help Sharon realize that it was she who conceptualized herself as of being enuretic, and she was responsible for the meaning she put into her own behavior. We looked at books with illustrations of the human body and of the bladder, and we discussed the brain and its role:

Therapist: Could you stand up please?
Sharon: Sure (standing up).
T: How did you do that?
S: What do you mean?
T: What made you stand up? From what you already learned about the brain.
S: Oh, yes, the brain commanded me to stand up.

At that point we talked about the way the brain is responsible for every one of our behaviors and about the connection between the brain and the body. Sharon was told about the differences between automatic, unmediated commands and mediated commands. As a homework assignment, she was asked to read material about the brain and the bladder and to try to observe her own behavior to determine commands the brain sends.

During the next few sessions, Sharon was helped to accept responsibility by learning to change her brain's commands. She practiced identifying automatic thoughts and using self-talk and self-recording to change unmediated thoughts into mediated ones. Various props were used such as plastic bags, to show how the bladder fills, and illustrations of the bladder and brain. Sharon was challenged to identify other automatic responses she had (e.g. being disruptive in the classroom, not doing her homework) and to change them into mediated thoughts. Daily, she charted one example of an automatic command that she was accustomed to performing and her plan for stopping and modifying this command. For example, discussing her eating habits, she mentioned that many times she found herself opening the refrigerator without even paying attention to the fact she was doing so, or without even being sure she wanted to eat. Sharon was helped to develop internal dialogues for self-instruction. In the case of the food, she decided to stop and ask herself: "Am I hungry now?" In another example, she mentioned how many times she left a room without being sure if she had turned off the light and therefore needed to return. She decided to purposely tell herself before leaving the room: "I'm going to turn the light off now." When asked to try changing the automatic response of bedwetting into self-restraint or awakening, Sharon said she felt she already knew how to do this.

In order to help Sharon understand how she could have her brain give the command to become dry, we practiced two therapist-generated metaphors, as differentiated from client-generated metaphors (Kopp, 1995). The former are introduced by the therapist in order to demonstrate, explain, or clarify some ideas in other than cognitive-verbal language. It is assumed that everyone's life is structured like a story, and that one's entire biographical tradition is based on that story. Transforming the story into metaphorical language can enhance understanding (Lakoff & Johnson, 1980). The first metaphor I introduced consisted of playing soldiers. I acted as commander and she needed to obey me. Practice of this metaphor served to clarify the way the brain commands the bladder to empty or to restrain. The second metaphor aimed to demonstrate how the automatic command could be changed. I asked her to draw a river. As she drew it, I asked her to note in which direction the river was flowing.

Therapist: Now, let's assume that I want to change the direction of the river's flow. What should I do?

Sharon: Build a dam.

T: Okay, I built a dam. Now, the river is flowing in all directions, but I want it to go to the opposite direction of how we began.

S: Well, then, you need to dig a tunnel.

T: O.K. Look, here is a new tunnel and a dam. The old tunnel reflects the brain's old command to wet the bed. The new tunnel is the new command to stay dry. Now let's point out where we are on the picture. You see, it seems as if you already dug a new tunnel, because four to five nights a week you stay dry, which means you are able to give new commands. You also built a dam, because on those nights it seems as if you are able to stop the old command to urinate. However, the wall of the dam is not tall enough, so some of the water succeeds in washing over it. How about if this week your assignment will be to deepen the tunnel and build a higher wall?

SCIM module 3: Attentional focus. While focusing on her wish to get rid of the enuresis, Sharon was not aware of her own internal sensations, neither was she ready to accept her feelings and internal stimuli. In order to learn to control her bladder, Sharon needed to direct her attention and focus on her internal stimuli. She had to learn to increase sensitivity to inner sensations, especially to the pressure of the bladder. A functional relationship exists between the size of the bladder and enuresis. A small bladder fills up quickly, and the signals it sends are less clear than those of a larger bladder (Fielding, 1980). In this stage, sensitivity to internal stimuli in general (e.g. the sensations of hunger, tiredness, etc.) and to the sensations of the bladder in particular, was increased. Sharon was asked to report her sensations in general (e.g. heartbeat, pulsation in the stomach, reception of noises, etc.) and her bladder pressure. As suggested in constructivist therapy, experiencing and exploration are very important for one's well-being. Sharon had to practice retention control exercises, both for enlarging the bladder and to increase sensitivity to internal stimuli. She was asked to practice restraining urination during the day and to concentrate on the ensuing sensations. Sharon's parents were instructed to ask her why she was going to the toilet, what did she feel, and where in the body the sensation was located. She learned to identify the specific physical sensation that occurred when she could not withhold any longer and must urinate.

To illustrate this, we went to the sink, and I took a plastic bag. I wanted to demonstrate to her how, when the bag is full of water, I need to close my fingers and hand tightly around the opening, if I want the water to remain inside while I turn the bag upside down.

By that time (about six weeks from the beginning of treatment), Sharon had decreased the frequency of wetting to about one to two nights a week.

SCIM module 4: Self-control exercises. In the fourth module, we worked on imparting self-control skills and techniques. First, Sharon was trained to gain physical control, and then she was trained to acquire control over emotions, thinking, and behavior. Techniques included the use of self-monitoring and assessment, self-instruction and self-reinforcement, imagery, and problem solving. For practice, she exercised self-control in day-to-day activities through homework assignments: to stop talking when she wanted to say something, to stop in the middle of playing or crying, and to stop drinking when thirsty or eating when hungry. Sharon was instructed to continue the physical exercises even when she felt tired or experienced some other difficulty. We used self-imagination as well as learning about the role of expectancies in behavior change:

Therapist: You have successfully decreased your wetting nights. Still, there are nights when you wet the bed. How do you explain this?

Sharon: I can't stop myself from wetting the bed.

T: You say that you can't control yourself. Is this the case all of the time?

S: Yes.

T: (I decided to use the fact that for the first time, Sharon had gone on an overnight school trip.) Two weeks ago you went for a trip with your class. Did you wet there?

S: Are you crazy? That would embarrass me terribly.

T: So what did you do?

S: I tried very hard and I succeeded.

T: Exactly! You see, when you think that it's important for you, you can control yourself. Now, imagine that your parents promise to give you the new compact disk set you desire so badly if you don't wet the bed. Would you succeed in doing it?

S: Sure I would.

T: You see, whenever it's important for you, if you're either afraid of being punished (having your friends notice that you wet the bed) or if you wish to gain something (a compact disk set), you put in more effort and succeed in staying dry. Doesn't that mean you can control your enuresis when it's important?

S: Maybe. I'm not sure.

T: How about us checking this out by you imagining every night for the next week that you will get that disk player you want if you stay dry, and putting in as much effort as you can?

S: I'll try.

As a homework assignment she was asked to keep a nightly chart predicting her enuresis for that night ("Do I believe I can stay dry or not?"). Every morning she had to chart if her prediction was accurate or not ("Did I succeed in staying dry?"). Then we talked about the link between her belief and her behavior, and the way the prediction can serve as a command to stay dry or wet. As she progressed, her nightly self-predictions more frequently became: "I am sure I will be dry." As she started believing in her ability to become dry, she was dry more and more often.

Throughout the whole process of change, Sharon was asked to use self-recording, self-evaluation, and self-reinforcement. Gradually, she could increase her self-confidence. She was asked to write down a positive self-evaluation every morning and she wrote things like:

I am 1000!
Well done!
I knew I could!
I'm proud of myself!

It seemed as if Sharon already knew how to be dry, and it was only a matter of time and practice until she completely overcome this problem.

After Sharon maintained three consecutive dry weeks, we terminated therapy. It was time to evaluate the treatment outcomes and move to a maintenance stage of intervention.

Phase 5 of Decision Making: Evaluating Sharon at the End of Therapy and Maintaining Treatment Outcomes

Evaluation. In line with the goal of Sharon's therapy, to decrease her enuretic behavior (see Table 4.8), two sources of information contributed to the evaluation of Sharon's treatment outcomes: parental reports and Sharon's charts. As described in the beginning of this chapter, Sharon's parents reported that she was very spoiled, did not take responsibility for her wetting, and did not cope independently. At the time of the referral, they took responsibility for cleaning her room and bed, and for handling her wetting altogether. During the last session, the parents reported: "It seems as if Sharon has grown up suddenly!" Sharon was taking responsibility for her own behavior, and the parents no longer had to deal with cleaning her bed, washing the laundry, or reminding her to go empty herself before going to sleep. Also, Sharon started behaving more independently in making decisions, in taking on specific chores in the family, and in going out and getting more involved with peer activities.

The second source of information consisted of Sharon's own charts on her wetting pattern. At the beginning of treatment, Sharon would wet the bed between five to six nights a week. Looking at her charts in the last four weeks of therapy showed that Sharon was dry.

Maintenance. As we entered the follow-up stage, we held one session every three weeks with Sharon and her parents, in line with the contact frequency outlined in Table 4.9.

One of the main foci of this stage was relapse prevention. Regression often occurs because, as one regresses, one tends to lose confidence in the ability to control the situation, and then a chain of regressions occurs. At this stage, Sharon was cautioned to regard any case of bedwetting as a predictable incidental event rather than a regression and a failure in achieving her target. She progressed wonderfully; however, I was expecting relapses to happen, and I was afraid it might be difficult for her to continue putting in efforts over a long period of time, especially if she regressed. Therefore, we redefined relapse as a necessary step toward a greater achievement, as the gap between two mountains that one faces while climbing up. I illustrated it to her by drawing a good circle and a bad circle. The good circle means that there is a connection between success, confidence, and efforts. As one succeeds one feels better, and then wishes to put in more effort, which results in more success. However, there is also the bad circle, which means that as one fails, one feels bad, loses confidence, and does not put in much effort, which causes another failure.

We talked about the fact that as Sharon regressed she became very disappointed and gave up investing efforts; therefore, she started wetting the bed more and more. The target therefore was while relapsing to tell herself: "Well, it is too bad I wet the bed, but I know how to overcome it, so tomorrow I will be dry again." She was cautioned to put in even more efforts at the time of relapse in order to remain in the "good circle."

The maintenance techniques focused on overlearning and relapse prevention, whereby Sharon was gradually instructed to cease earlier limitations on her bedtime behavior, and to begin drinking before bed, going to bed without emptying herself in the toilet first, going to sleep at whatever time she chose, etc. She was advised to keep up her charts, and the follow-up sessions served as an incentive to persevere in recording despite her continued success.

After three months of being dry, the follow-up stage was terminated. Sharon stayed dry even when she went to sleep late, drank before going to sleep, or forgot to empty herself before going to bed. The charts emphasized the change in her wetting behavior and showed that Sharon was dry and did not regress. Follow-up by telephone revealed that Sharon stayed dry.

11

Oppositional Defiant Disorder

LITERATURE REVIEW

The problem of aggressive behavior in children is addressed in the *DSM-IV* (American Psychiatric Association, 1994) under the general category of "attention-deficit/hyperactive and disruptive disorders," which includes conduct disorder, oppositional defiant disorder, disruptive behavior, and attention-deficit/hyperactive disorder. The most frequently used definitions are conduct disorder and oppositional defiant disorder.

In trying to differentiate between them, conduct disorder is defined as children who engage in a persistent pattern of behavior that violates either the basic rights of others or major age-appropriate societal norms or rules (American Psychiatric Association, 1994). A less severe disorder, but one that might presage conduct disorder, is oppositional defiant disorder (ODD) (Scotti et al., 1998). ODD involves a recurrent pattern of negativistic, defiant, disobedient, and hostile behavior toward authority figures. It should last at least 6 months, during which four or more of the following are present: often loses temper; often argues with adults; often actively defies or refuses to comply with adults' requests or rules; often deliberately annoys people; often blames others for his or her mistakes or misbehavior; is often touchy or easily annoyed by others; is often angry and resentful; and/or is often spiteful or vindictive (DSM-IV, American Psychiatric Association, 1994). Other DSM-IV criteria include clinically significant impairment in social, academic, or occupational functioning that stems from the disturbance in behavior, and the stipulation that the child's oppositional behavior does not occur exclusively during the course of a psychotic or mood disorder. Differential diagnosis of ODD requires that criteria should not be met for either conduct disorder (aggression toward people or animals, destruction of property, a pattern of theft or deceit) or antisocial personality disorder (over age 18).

This said, the lines between disruptive, oppositional defiant, and conduct disorders are often blurred, with definitions and groupings used interchangeably. Inconsistency and different views exist with regard to identifying those children who should be diagnosed with each of the separate disorders. Part of the complexity in achieving coherent, distinct definitions may be rooted in the extremely broad range of acting-out, undercontrolled, and externalizing behaviors (Achenbach, 1985, 1993; Kazdin, 1987, 1998; Kazdin et al., 1987) evidenced by such children. Their behaviors include high rates of noncompliance and defiance in response to teacher requests, aggressiveness, cruelty toward peers, destructive acts, smart talk, lying, stealing, running away, cheating, and many more. Usually, children with disruptive behavior disorders also present comorbidity with learning difficulties, hyperactive and impulsive disorders, anger, anxiety, and depression. It is notably difficult to determine the etiological interrelations between the different comorbid childhood behaviors.

To avoid confusion, in the present chapter, I will generally refer to ODD when addressing children with various degrees of aggressive behavior disorders.

Regardless of diagnostic labels, the effects of aggressive behavior disorders constitute a major social problem and one of the most frequent reasons for children's referrals (Kazdin et al., 1990). Behavioral disorders have a relatively poor long-term prognosis and are transmitted across generations (Kazdin, 1998). Estimates have indicated that children's disruptive, oppositional, and conduct disorders encompass from one-third to one-half of all child and adolescent clinic referrals (Herbert, 1987; Webster-Stratton, 1993). The prevalence of these problems is 6–16% among boys and 2–9% among girls in the regular population (Webster-Stratton, 1993). ODD is very frequent among school aged children. Teachers usually encounter at least two or more children in their classrooms each year exhibiting persistent patterns of disruptive and antisocial behavior (Webster-Stratton, 1993). This comprises a social disorder at the focus of public interest.

For assessment purposes and to select optimal treatment techniques, researchers have attempted to conceptualize these undercontrolled, aggressive behaviors in several ways. Some differentiate between physically aggressive and verbally aggressive behavior, and some discriminate reactive from proactive behavior. Some trace a dynamic process that starts as quiet negativism, develops into disruptive disorders and ODD, and then continues to evolve into conduct and antisocial disorders.

No clear explanation or theory exists to elucidate the development of anger or violent behavior. It is difficult to explain why one child develops adaptive behavior while another develops aggressive behavior. Kazdin (1998) stated that the main problem in treating ODD lies in the fact that there is no standard, consistent explanation to link theory, assessment, diagnosis, treatment, and evaluation.

Therefore, it is a complex task to determine systematic goals for intervention or effective data based methods for changing this problem.

Bandura and colleagues (2001) recently proposed a theoretical explanation for the development of aggressive behavior. They conceptualized behavior as the capacity to exercise some measure of control over one's thought processes, motivation, affect, and actions, which all operate through mechanisms of personal agency. The most crucial mechanism is the self-efficacy mechanism (Bandura, 1997). These authors claimed that unless people believe they can bring about desired outcomes and forestall undesired ones by their actions, they have little incentive to act or to persevere in the face of difficulties and adversities.

Bandura and his colleagues (2001) suggested that aggressive behavior results from three main components: academic efficacy, social efficacy, and self-regulatory efficacy. These three components are interlinked and influence one another. All three are related to prosocial behavior as well as moral disengagement. Likewise, they are all associated with ruminative affectivity and therefore may result in transgressive behavior. According to this theory, aggressive behavior could be prevented if the child is involved in academic learning in a caring school that challenges children to achieve and that explicitly teaches both prosocial peer involvement as well as personal self-efficacy (Bandura et al., 2001).

No matter if the children exhibit physical or verbal aggressiveness, whether it is proactive or reactive, they usually exhibit a negative, hostile way of looking at the world and their place in it. Their thoughts are generally very rigid and distorted, and their emotional repertoire is often colored by anger, irritability, and animosity.

Clearly, a large gap exists between the definition of diagnostic criteria, which is based on behavior, and the theorized characteristics of externalizing children, which include cognitive and affective features. The clinical definition focuses on the acting-out behavior, whereas the theoretical explanation emphasizes acting-in features such as thinking style and feelings.

Treatment

The past three decades have seen a progressive advancement of behavioral technology for the remediation of childhood conduct disorders and ODD (Scotti et al., 1998). Many different treatments have been applied to conduct-disordered youth including psychotherapy; pharmacotherapy; psychosurgery; home, school, and community based programs; residential and hospital treatments; and social services (Kazdin, 1998). Of the 230 documented psychotherapies available for children and adolescence (Kazdin, 1988a), the vast majority has not been examined empirically. Kazdin stated that a large variety of treatments are conducted with aggressive children, where dynamic therapy is the most popular despite its lower effectiveness than other methods. Cognitively based treatments have been found to significantly reduce aggressiveness at home, at school, and in the community (Bailey, 1998).

Kazdin (1998) mentioned three kinds of promising treatment programs to address children who evidence aggressive behavior: functional family therapy, parent counseling, and cognitive problem-solving models. These programs each offer some theoretical rationale to explicate how the dysfunction comes about and how treatment redresses the dysfunction. Basic research supports each program's conceptualization, and outcome data for each have shown effective change.

Functional family therapy. This integrative approach to treatment relies on systems, behavioral, and cognitive views of dysfunction (Alexander et al., 1994). Clinical problems are conceptualized in terms of the functions they serve in the family as a system, as well as for individual family members. Maladaptive processes within the family are considered to preclude a more direct means of fulfilling these functions. The goal of treatment is to alter interaction and communication patterns in such a way as to foster more adaptive functioning. Treatment is also based on learning theory and focuses on specific stimuli and responses that can be used to produce change.

Functional family therapy requires that the family see the clinical problem in light of the relational function it serves within the family (Kazdin, 1998). The therapist points out interdependencies and contingencies among the family members in their day to day functioning and with specific reference to the problem. The main goal of therapy is to increase reciprocity and positive reinforcement among family members, to establish clear communication, and to help improve family relationships.

Relatively few outcome studies have evaluated the family functioning method (Alexander et al., 1994). However, the controlled studies that have been conducted showed it to surpass the effectiveness of client centered family groups and of psychodynamically oriented family therapy (Kazdin, 1998).

Parent counseling. Parent treatment programs are multifarious. In parent management training, the therapist teaches parents to use specific procedures that alter their child's behavior at home and their interaction with the child, promoting prosocial behavior, and decreasing deviant behavior (Kazdin, 1998). A common intervention used to address the excessive behavior of children with ODD and conduct disorders involves teaching parents to apply procedures that change the environmental variables influencing their child's behavior. Such programs are based on the assumption that parental skills deficits are contributing factors to the development and maintenance of child behavior problems (Webster-Stratton, 1993). The aim of such programs is to indirectly change child behavior by directly changing parenting behavior (Patterson, 1982). Although a wealth of parent-training packages exist, few have been empirically studied. Among them, the most popular and well studied are those proposed by Forehand and McMahon (1981), Patterson (1976, 1982), and Webster-Stratton (1982).

The most well known parent-training program, coercion, was developed by Patterson (1982). Coercion refers to deviant behavior on the part of one person (the child) that is rewarded by another person (the parent). Aggressive children are inadvertently rewarded for their aggressive interactions and their escalation of coercive behaviors, as part of the discipline practices that sustain aggressive behavior. The critical role of parent–child discipline practices has been supported by correlational research, which related specific discipline practices to children's antisocial behavior (Kazdin, 1998).

In general, parent training is characterized by five main components (Bailey, 1998):

1. Parents are taught how to pinpoint the problem behaviors and track them at home, for example, recording compliance versus noncompliance.
2. Parents are taught reinforcement techniques, for example, praise, point systems, and giving treats and rewards.
3. When parents see their children behaving inappropriately, they learn to apply a mild consequence or a short-term deprivation of privileges, for example, one hour loss of television time or bike use.
4. Parents are taught to monitor their children at all times, even when they are away from home. This involves parents knowing where their children are at all times, what they are doing, and when they will be returning home.
5. Finally, the parents are taught problem-solving and negotiating strategies. They also become increasingly responsible for designing their own programs.

Cognitive problem-solving techniques. The rationale for applying individual interventions in cases of ODD and conduct disorders is based on the range of cognitive deficits and distortions evidenced by these children (Bailey, 1998; Crick & Dodge, 1994). These children recall high rates of hostile cues in social situations, attend to few cues when interpreting the meaning of others' behavior, and attribute the behavior of others to hostile intentions when in ambiguous situations. When they are in contact with other aggressive children, they tend to underestimate their own level of aggression.

Cognitive problem-solving skills training consist of developing interpersonal cognitive problem-solving skills. Several characteristics are usually common to the various treatments applied for children with ODD. First, the way children approach situations is emphasized, particularly the thought processes in which the child engages that guide responses to interpersonal situations. Children are taught to engage in a step-by-step approach. Second, the behaviors selected by the child in interpersonal situations are targeted. Prosocial behaviors are fostered as part of the problem-solving process. Third, the treatment utilizes structured tasks involving games, academic activities, and stories. Over the course of treatment, the cognitive problem-solving skills are increasingly applied to real life situations. Fourth, the therapist plays an active role in treatment. Finally, treatment usually combines several different procedures including modeling and practice exercises.

Studies have shown that this method is effective for reducing aggressive behavior (Durlak et al., 1991) both in outpatient and inpatient clinics (Kazdin, 1994b; Kendall, 1993). Intervention studies have shown that teaching a child to refrain from aggressive cognitions, and to emphasize alternative social cognitions, successfully decreases actual aggressive behavior

Cognitive and behavioral interventions have commonly been directed toward imparting aggressive children with deficient skills. Among the individual cognitive therapies, one of the most popular techniques for reducing ODD and conduct disorders is the application of social skills training. Such programs incorporate constant reinforcements of prosocial behavior and discussions of antisocial behavior (Bailey, 1998), with training to improve social relationships via role-play, observation, modeling, and practicing techniques.

The following case study will illustrate how cognitive constructivist treatment can address the need to apply self-control skills to an adolescent suffering from ODD.

TREATING GUY: AN ADOLESCENT WITH OPPOSITIONAL DEFIANT DISORDER

First Session with Guy and His Parents

As Guy and his parents entered my clinic, it was obvious to me that something had been going on between them before they came in, and they were still under its impression. Tension and anger hung in the air before they even spoke. Usually, I ask the child to introduce me to the parents. I am interesting in watching what the child says, how he or she presents the problem, and how the parents react. However, this time, it was very difficult to start talking with this family, so after introducing myself, I asked them to tell me what brought them to my office, turning specifically to Guy. He refused to talk with me, sitting with his eyes lowered toward the floor, on the opposite side of the room from his parents. I was quiet for a few minutes, and then the mother shouted out: "That's it. I can't take this anymore! I am sick and tired of getting phone calls from his school. If he can't change, he'll have to leave home. This time, I'll send him off to a school far away!" Guy barked in reply: "This time it wasn't my fault. I know the teacher hates me. She's lying. You never listen to me, only to them. That's it, I'm leaving. There's no reason for me to stay here." He stood up, intending to leave the room, and I told him: "I see you're very angry. I understand that you feel that everyone is turning against you. Maybe you're right, but if you leave now, we won't be able to see if you're right. Will you sit down and help me understand what's going on here? You don't have to come back again, if you don't want to. But since you're already here, let's use the time we have, and talk about it." Guy looked at me, and then sat down, saying, "Okay, but I'm not coming here again."

I knew, based on my prior telephone call from the mother, that she and her husband were furious because Guy had been involved in a fight, and they had been asked to come to school and take him home. He was suspended from school for 3 days, and the school principal said she would only accept Guy back to school if he started therapy.

A few minutes later, as Guy sat back down, I asked him to introduce all of his family members to me, and he complied. First, he said: "I'm not talking about them! Let them introduce themselves if they want to. I don't care!" Then he started to describe himself. He was 14 years of age and the middle child of three. He had an older brother aged 17, who was about to graduate high school and join the army. He also had a younger sister aged 12, who attended the same junior high school where he studied. He then pointed to his parents and said: "If you want to know about them, ask them!" The father took over and continued. He said he was a technician in a telephone company, and the mother was a secretary.

The mother then told me that Guy's two siblings were good students, had good friends, and had no problems in school, in contrast to their brother Guy, who was always getting into fights and into trouble. Ever since he was in kindergarten, she continued, Guy was involved in fighting. Usually he did not start fights, but whenever someone picked on him or laughed at him, he would respond in a very exaggerated way. As the mother talked, Guy sat with his head down, making all kinds of angry gestures as if in reply to his mother's narrative. He shook his head, cursed under his breath, and sometimes turned his fists toward his mother.

The mother said that Guy was a smart boy and a good student. As Guy heard this, he asked: "Oh, so you also remember some good things, huh? What happened to you? Are you trying to impress Tammie?" The mother continued saying that, despite his impulsive behavior over many years, he was still very popular among his friends, and received good grades. She described him as a handsome, nice child with a good sense of humor and a great verbal ability. He could be very convincing when he explained how others always caused him to react as he did, and why it was not his fault. The teachers used to forgive him, because they appreciated his intelligence. He was so persuasive that it was very difficult to argue with him. However, lately, she continued, his behavior had become so disturbing that the teachers had lost their patience, he had begun to receive lower grades, and his friends were not putting up with his aggravations any longer. At home, Guy was constantly at odds with his parents, arguing to try to reverse his parents' decisions and make them do what he wanted. They felt they no longer had the patience or energy to continue arguing with him. The mother said she was exhausted. The father was bothered by his behavior as well, but said that he believed it would disappear in time, because "Guy is a smart boy, and one day he'll grow up, understand, and change his behavior." The parents had come to me with Guy because they did not see any other solution, and were being forced by the school to start therapy.

Guy seemed to be very angry and repeated that he would not come anymore. He did not need therapy, and if the parents wanted therapy, they could come. I told Guy that maybe he was right. Maybe he was not the one who needed treatment, but rather his parents. I commented that it was very reasonable to assume that they needed supervision to learn how to handle him. But, I added, in order to know what was needed, I would have to meet with him at least one time, to find out what the problem was. Guy agreed to come for one session, individually, but he emphasized that only once, and without his parents.

Assessing Guy

Adolescents are generally assessed using self-report and family self-reports (see Table 4.3). However, the oppositional nature of Guy's problem (see the treatment goal of "decreasing behavior" on Table 4.2) contraindicated a heavy reliance on self-reports. Children suffering from defiant, aggressive, undercontrolled behavior usually view others as the main cause for their behavior and do not take responsibility upon themselves. Thus, as I described in Chapter 1, children's self-reports are not a reliable source regarding their own acting-out or externalizing behaviors, in comparison with parents' and teachers' reports of such conduct.

I therefore decided to assess Guy first by interviewing both his parents and his teacher, and by obtaining their impressions about his behavior via a standardized behavior questionnaire. With the parents' permission, I administered the Child Behavior Checklist (Achenbach & Edelbrock, 1983) separately with the teacher and with both parents. Using the part of the scale related to aggressive behavior, Guy was found to be aggressive by both the parents' and the teacher's questionnaires.

In addition, I thought it would be important to learn about Guy's own perspective through an interview with him and to observe his behavior directly in sessions conducted with his parents, or with me individually. I met with Guy the following week. I told him that I appreciated the fact that he came, and that it was important for me to learn what he thought, how he felt, and what changes his parents needed to make.

I asked Guy to explain to me what the problem was, why he acted as he did, and what his future plans were. Guy explained that the situation was not his fault. Children were always picking on him and laughing at him, and they made him angry. His narrative could be understood in terms of "them" versus "me." "Them" were the others in his life: parents, teachers, children. "They" never understood him, and always blamed him. Only he would be punished, not them. They expected him to behave differently, but they never understood him.

Guy talked repeatedly about the injustice of the world, and the fact that the world was unfair and unjust. Each person had to fight for himself, and there was no reason to be good in this world, because good people always lose. As proof, he offered both his parents. They were not assertive, they were too good, and they lost out. His mother did not receive as much inheritance as her brothers, when her parents died, because she was too good and always gave in. His father failed to get a promotion at work because he did not know how to fight for it, and other employees were always getting promoted instead of him. Guy said he was going to be different. He wanted to know how to fight for himself and get what he wanted. It was clear that Guy held very rigid, negative beliefs and thoughts about the world. His range of emotional expression was limited to anger, hostility, or gloating at another's failure. He could not talk about things that made him happy, excited, or amused, unless these were related to other people's mistakes or suffering. In discussing his behavior, he always viewed others at the root of his actions, consistently blaming others for his arguments or fights.

I felt he was enjoying the attention he received from me, and I was able to obtain his agreement to continue coming, under the condition that he came alone, without his parents. He said he agreed to come because he wanted to persuade me that he was right and his parents were wrong.

Phase 1 of Decision Making: Does Guy Need Therapy or Not?

The decision of whether or not Guy should be treated was based, first of all, on problem variables (see Table 4.1). Guy's behavior clearly met the clinical diagnostic criteria for ODD (*DSM-IV*, American Psychiatric Association, 1994). He constantly engaged in a persistent pattern of behavior (hitting, fistfights, arguing, cursing, laughing at others, damaging their belongings) that violated the basic rights of others. Guy evidenced all the criteria of the negativistic, defiant, disobedient, and hostile behaviors specified in the *DSM-IV*, toward authority figures at home and at school (Scotti et al., 1998). Guy was hot-tempered, argumentative, actively defiant, deliberately annoying, easily irritated, angry, resentful, spiteful, vindictive, and blamed others for his misbehavior. This behavior pattern was lifelong, but had worsened over the last 4 months. It was unlikely to improve on its own, and this deterioration posed a risk to him academically as well as socially.

In terms of developmental variables, adolescents often exhibit disobedient behavior, as part of their normal maturation processes. Rebellion and alienation from parents oftentimes are part and parcel of teenagers' attempts to establish a separate identity and forge an independent existence in the world. However, Guy's behavior was, by all accounts, much more extreme, deviating significantly from his age and sex group and his environmental surroundings. The school even viewed the problem as severe enough to warrant immediate intervention.

In examining child and family variables, aggressive children do not usually present personal motivation for change. They view themselves as strong human beings who control the environment. Instead, parents and teachers are generally those who instigate a referral for treatment. Correspondingly, in Guy's case, the school and his parents were the most highly motivated figures for change, much more than Guy himself. However, based on Kanfer and Schefft (1988), I believe that everyone has motivation. We need only to uncover what they are motivated toward. I thought I could increase Guy's motivation for therapy by focusing on improving his peer relationships and by talking about "getting his parents off his back."

One question to ask in evaluating child and family variables involves emotional states. Guy's parents were in a very difficult emotional state. They were the main individuals suffering from the situation. Guy did not feel he was suffering. Actually, he sensed himself to be at the center of attention, and he felt strong and able to extensively influence and even control his environment. He saw no reason to give up that control.

Relating to treatment variables, prognostically, ODD is a behavior that can be changed. However, it can be more easily changed by working with the environment than by working only individually with the child. Little chance existed for Guy's spontaneous recovery, due to the fact that his problem had only worsened over the years and in light of his lack of motivation to give up the sense of power he gained from his behavior. A good likelihood for change via treatment could be expected, if the school and the parents complied with therapeutic supervision.

Guy was an intelligent boy and had the capacity to establish good interpersonal relationships, as manifested in the fact that, despite his annoying and antagonistic behavior, Guy was still liked among his teachers and friends. I therefore believed I could establish a good therapeutic relationship with him.

Phase 2 of Decision Making: Classifying Guy's Referral and Goals for Change

Clearly, the disobedient, aggressive conduct presented at Guy's referral could be classified as the first of the four types of childhood behavior problems: an acting-out, undercontrolled behavior problem obviously needing reduction (see Table 4.2). The goal for Guy's treatment was defined as decreasing his negativism, defiance, and oppositional behavior. In addition, it was important to relate to the second goal of referral: Increasing a behavior for helping Guy improve his prosocial behavior.

Guy's problem was also considered in light of the developmental tasks confronting adolescents his age (see Table 4.3). At age 14, Guy seemed to evidence difficulties in all aspects of adolescent development. His defiant behavior reflected a maladaptive pattern of separating from his parents; deficits in the process of establishing a healthy individualization or any autonomy for himself that did not rely on aggressive or antisocial means; and difficulties in family interaction. He exhibited striking deficiencies in self-control at home and at school. He was formulating an identity based on an antagonistic attitude toward the world and his place in it, typified by a bitter and resentful emotional life.

Phases 3 of Decision Making: Selecting Who Should Be Treated

To determine the therapeutic setting, Guy's problem type and developmental stage were considered. Treatment of ODD, a behavior that must be decreased, is usually directed toward the environment (see Table 4.5). This disorder may be changed primarily or exclusively by training the environment in how to reinforce positive behavior and punish or avoid unwanted behavior. Guy's problematic interactions at home and at school plainly suggested the urgency of supervision for Guy's parents and teachers.

Moreover, largely in view of the crucial developmental task of formulating a healthy identity at his age (see Table 4.4), I determined that Guy must also be treated individually. The risk was high that Guy, who already experienced continually hostile emotions and held rigidly negative beliefs about the world and himself, might integrate these cognitions and affects into his developing identity, thus reducing the likelihood that he could positively adjust to society in the future. Guy's developmental stage, as well as the referral goal of increasing Guy's prosocial behavior and ability to express positive emotions (Table 4.5), were conducive to treating him individually. Adolescents can enjoy individual therapy and are usually treated alone or, at times, within the family.

Thus, in combining the two aforementioned considerations, I determined to treat Guy individually and to supervise his parents and his teacher.

Phase 4 of Decision Making: Selecting Guy's Optimal Treatment Modes

Both Guy's developmental stage and problem area highlighted the necessity of verbally training Guy and his parents in methods to decrease his recalcitrant behavior and improve his prosocial behavior. Disobedient behavior is a problem that can better be addressed by behavioral and cognitive methods, and less by constructivist methods. This was true in Guy's case because the major need was to directly impart Guy with skills for behavior change. Guy's type of disorder, one requiring a decrease in behavior, particularly accentuated the suitability of verbal therapy (see Table 4.7). Guy's aims in therapy would be to learn to change his thoughts, emotions, and behaviors and, mainly, to acquire problem-solving skills that would alter his habitual responses. However, in treating Guy's emotional problems (increasing awareness to internal stimuli, learning to express positive as well as negative emotions) and helping him gain prosocial skills, constructivist therapy would be the treatment of choice. I felt I needed to be creative in order to mobilize Guy's motivation, overcome his rejection, and get him to comply with therapy assignments. This, as well as the need to increase emotional and prosocial behaviors, necessitated the use of indirect methods such as imagery (see Table 4.7).

As a 14-year-old boy, Guy might reject drawing or painting techniques as too childish. He was intelligent and strongly relied on that shrewdness as a means for achieving his goals. Hence, therapy could mobilize these strengths in order to change his unwanted behavior: his ability to talk, persuade others, and conduct verbal communication. His developmental stage suggested the need for verbal therapy (see Table 4.6).

All of the above phases of consideration led easily to the decision that Guy's case warranted treatment, and that both he individually and his environment required intervention. In sum, Guy's treatment would have three main goals: to impart skills to the teacher that could cease Guy's disobedient behavior; to train the parents in techniques that reinforce desired behavior and decrease noncompliant behavior; and to impart Guy himself with self-control skills. Those skills could help him modify his negative attitudes toward the world, help him express positive emotion, and teach him to handle better and to express in a more acceptable way his negative emotions, mainly his anger. Also, he needed to be trained in problem-solving skills to decrease his aggressive behavior. Therapy would have a mostly verbal cognitive focus, and would address internal components as well as social and environmental issues.

The Intervention Process

The preliminary contract included Guy and his parents. We agreed on three main issues: the need to supervise the teacher, the need to train the parents, and the need to treat Guy. All treatment modes were carried out in parallel, at the same time.

Supervising the Teacher

The parents gave their permission to share the treatment program with Guy's homeroom teacher and to supervise her. I initially went to school to talk with her, and then we agreed on weekly telephone calls.

At first, it was difficult to persuade Guy's teacher that there was a need for her to change how she related to him. She believed that by talking to Guy, explaining what was right and what was wrong, and not punishing him, he would finally understand how to behave, because he was actually a nice, smart boy. It took a while for her to understand that Guy was actually relying upon this attitude of hers, and that, as long as he went unpunished and received so much attention, he would not change his behavior.

We decided on gradual goals for change and on techniques to reinforce his behavior. The first problem the teacher raised was Guy's jokes. Guy would make quips during the lessons, causing his classmates to burst out in laughter, and thus disrupting her teaching. We decided that every morning she would give Guy 5 minutes to tell jokes but then ask him to refrain from humorous interference for the rest of the day. Whenever he succeeded, she could give him another 5 minutes near the end of the day, as reinforcement. However, if he started interrupting her in the middle of class, she would ignore him and continue talking.

It was very difficult for the teacher to comply with this plan, and two weeks passed before she was able to begin implementing it consistently. Then, it took about two more weeks before Guy complied and stopped interrupting in the middle of class.

The second problem she noted was Guy's tendency to call out his answers to her questions in class whenever he wished, without raising his hand. Again, I directed her to make a contract with Guy, that she would try and ask him whenever he raised his hand and then praise him loudly. However, if he shouted out the answer, she would ignore him and let another child answer, even if his answer was correct. We also decided that if Guy complied, she would send a note to his parents telling them about Guy's obedience and his wonderful answers in class. As treatment progressed, we decided to target additional, similar goals, such as refraining from standing up in the middle of a lesson, avoiding hitting children during recess, restraining the urge to take other children's supplies, and so on.

The punishments Guy most commonly received in school consisted of being sent to the principal when he was disruptive, being sent out of the class, and inviting his parents to the school. In my view, each of these punishments served as a reinforcement. Guy liked the principal, who used to tell him stories when he was sent to her office. In collaboration with the principal, we reframed this situation, and Guy was told he would go the principal to hear stories every week if he improved.

Similarly, being sent out of class was far from a punishment for Guy, who would go to the physical education teacher and help him out in his class. We involved the physical education teacher in the treatment program. Guy was permitted to join him only if Guy handed him a note from his homeroom teacher. At the same time, we made an agreement with Guy: Every week that he improved, he would get permission to skip one lesson and go help the sports teacher.

Finally, I thought that calling Guy's parents in the middle of the day, bringing them to school, or sending Guy home with them simply constituted another reinforcement of Guy's behavior. We agreed that the school would inform me, instead of the parents, when there was trouble. Guy would not be suspended from school as a punishment.

During the first week of intervention, Guy's behavior deteriorated. He disrupted the class much more. It was extremely difficult to persuade his teacher that Guy was testing her limits in this first stage and that we should proceed with the program as planned. I received calls from her every night and had to repeatedly encourage and support her to prevent her from giving up. After two weeks, a slight improvement in his behavior could be noted. After a month, the teacher could say that something was really starting to change. Guy had stopped interrupting in the middle of the lesson by telling jokes, and he no longer called out his answers indiscriminately. After the first month, we decided that he would begin meeting directly with the teacher once a week. She would reinforce him for his obedient behavior, and together they would decide on the next goal without my involvement.

Another initial difficulty I encountered in supervising the teacher was to help her understand the importance of focusing only on the targeted behaviors (e.g. joking, calling out answers) and not on other problematic issues. It was a challenge to persuade her that she should try to ignore the other disruptions. The teacher used to ask Guy questions like: "You were so good at stopping your jokes without permission, so why can't you also stop taking things from your friends?" I had to be very consistent and optimistic in guiding her to adhere to the program until they could gradually move on to other targets. I continued to make myself available as a resource for the teacher whenever she felt she needed consultation or was afraid of regression.

I continued supervising the teacher throughout the whole process of treating Guy. However, after the first two months, it seemed as if the teacher already understood the main principles of behavior change (e.g. deciding on a specific behavior, reinforcing Guy's achievement, ignoring his other disturbances, challenging his positive resources, and motivating him to continue progress), and she needed me less. Supervision calls became mainly a report about his progress, and reinforcing the teacher's behavior.

Counseling the Parents

Guy's parents had reached the point where they were so angered by his behavior that they immediately started shouting, lecturing, and punishing him for every little thing he did that did not comply with their wishes. Their responses were inconsistent, moving from punishment and anger, to deliberate attempts to ignore their son's behavior. These inconsistent reactions actually served as reinforcements for Guy's unwanted behavior. Moreover, because the parents had to leave work often to come to school, and much of the talk in the family surrounded his behavior, Guy had become the center of the family's attention, and he gained a sense of power from his behavior. All this had to be stopped in order to change his behavior.

During the first two sessions with Guy's parents, I taught them cognitive behavioral theory and techniques for behavior change. I also gave them two books to read about how to educate their children for self-control, and how to discipline their children. We talked about reinforcement, punishment methods, recording, self-evaluation, and paradoxical methods. I emphasized the importance of being consistent, adhering regularly to the program, and working together toward goals.

The first thing I asked them to do was to stop lecturing their son. I thought Guy had a precise understanding of the difference between right and wrong, and he would not benefit from lectures and explanations, which, indeed, would only reinforce his unwanted behavior. Like the teacher, the parents lacked a basic understanding that Guy needed clear, consistent limits on his behavior. Based on the misconception and the hope that Guy would act appropriately once he understood why and what he should be doing, the parents had continually explained things to him instead of punishing or limiting him. Guy capitalized on their forgiveness and simply continued his oppositional, defiant behavior. The more the parents forgave and understood, the worse his behavior became.

I asked them to monitor his behavior during the first two weeks and then to decide on the first two specific issues they wanted to address. I suggested we start with something small and easy that would be conducive to measurement. We wanted to be able to tell when it started and when it stopped when trying to change it.

The mother first selected the problem of Guy's loud interruptions in the middle of her conversations with friends or other family members. He would not stop his clamor unless she ceased talking and gave him what he wanted. We devised a plan whereby she would try to give Guy what he wanted when he waited for his turn, but she would act as if she did not hear him whenever he interrupted her in the middle of conversation. No matter what he wanted, he could not obtain it if he asked for it in a disruptive fashion. As expected, the mother's new behavior elicited a great deal of shouting and anger on Guy's part at first, but when she persevered, he began changing his behavior.

The next issues that the parents selected were for Guy to stop cursing and stop strewing his belongings all over the living room. The hardest thing to change was for Guy to stop picking on his siblings, and we left this for the end of therapy.

A great improvement appeared in Guy's behavior during the first two months of intervention, as both the teacher/school and the parents developed the ability to appropriately ignore him, give him positive reinforcements, and put limits on his behavior. Guy's aggressive, defiant behaviors had significantly changed via the common treatment mode for his disorder: teaching and changing the environment (Patterson, 1976, 1982).

Nevertheless, Guy's fatalistic, rigid thoughts about the world and his negative emotions did not change. His external demeanor was becoming increasingly appropriate in both his home and school environments; yet Guy continued to say that he was changing his behavior only in order to get what he wanted, and that he "would teach his parents and teachers who's really right." Although he stopped hitting his friends, he did not stop laughing at them or picking on them, and his social relationships did not improve. Now, Guy's parents and teacher said that he was not aggressive but was difficult to handle and made them angry. At this point, we focused mainly on the goals of decreasing Guy's destructive behavior and increasing his social skills.

Individual Therapy with Guy

Guy was treated using the SCIM training model described in Chapter 5, mainly via verbal therapy, by implementing social skills and problem solving methods, and with an additional focus on emotional issues.

SCIM module 1: Cognitive restructuring and redefinition. Guy kept blaming everyone but himself for his behavior. He tended to see others as the cause of his problems and did not take responsibility for his own behavior. The first module of the intervention aimed to change Guy's attributional style by teaching him that picking on other children, hitting, disrupting, and annoying others were behaviors that he himself was carrying out, and that it was his choice whether or not to act that way. Maybe he did not know how to act differently, or maybe he was afraid of losing control if he changed, but, regardless of the reasons, it was his decision and his alone. At that point, Guy objected to my interpretation, saying that: "It just happened," "Arguments took place," or "Children's belongings were broken." He was not yet able to use a first person voice (to say I broke, I argued, etc.) that would indicate acceptance of personal culpability.

Guy perceived himself as a strong person who was making the decisions in his life and who could control the others around him. I redefined his behavior as that of someone very weak who was controlled by others. He obviously disliked this reframing and tried to prove to me how strong he was. He explained how he could make the teacher angry and lose control, how children were afraid of him, and how he infuriated his parents. Repeatedly and consistently, I told him that really strong people do not have to hit or shout. They talk, and they expect others to do what they want because others will know that they are strong. I spelled out to Guy that, because he was weak and did not believe in himself, his only recourse was to make others fear him. Guy seemed to be angry with me, and kept threatening to leave treatment. However, I sensed that deep down he agreed with me, and he was not happy about his social situation. I felt he was not yet ready to admit that he was the cause of all the tumult in his life, and he certainly was not yet sure that he could change his behavior. Nevertheless, I could see that Guy's eyes and facial expression hinted at his curiosity and interest in what I was talking about.

I asked Guy to observe his own behavior over the week, and to observe his classmates to see which children were the ones whom most of the class followed, how they did it, who he saw as being strong, and how he would like to be strong. At the next session a week later, Guy came in and started talking again in the third person: "There were arguments in class …" "Things were happening … ." I kept asking him, smiling: "Things? They?" and eventually he spit out: "Well, okay, I, me, I! Are you satisfied now? I was talking, and no one was listening! Does that make you happy?" I said I was happy. Not because no one listened to him. That was probably very frustrating. But because I thought he was progressing. He was able to observe his own behavior, take responsibility, and talk about himself, and view what was going on around. Guy reported that he was very frustrated: When he talked, nobody paid attention to him, and that was why he needed to shout. I redefined this: Guy had taught the other children that he was so weak that they could make him shout and hit whenever they wanted. My redefinition of him as a weak rather than strong young person disturbed him greatly. He was angry and did not want to talk with me for the rest of the session. He then told me that he would prove to me how strong he was, and I answered quietly that a strong person is one who controls himself. Guy did not answer and left the room.

He arrived at the next session asking me, "What do I have to do to prove to you that I am strong?" I explained to him that strong people are those who decide how to act and then behave as they planned. He said, "Well, I am strong, and I can control myself and I will prove it to you, just to show you how wrong you are!" As the parents had learned, often the only successful way to enlist Guy's cooperation was to challenge him in a paradoxical way. Guy was not yet taking responsibility for his behavior or showing a wish to change it. However, it troubled him that I thought he was weak, and he was ready to do things just to prove me wrong. At that point, I settled for that.

To paradoxically challenge Guy, I remarked that I did not believe he could, at that stage, take responsibility for his own behavior, and certainly could not refrain from picking on other kids. However, I would like him to plan ahead that week, and to decide in advance who he was going to tease and when, and then to see if he could carry out what he had planned.

That week Guy invested a great deal of effort in improving his social behavior. He arrived at the next session very pleased with himself, reporting that he was behaving very well, had not been involved in arguments, and did not pick on anyone. He wanted me to admit that he could be strong and could take responsibility for his own behavior. I tried to help him talk about how different his feelings might be that week, when his parents were not getting angry reports from the teacher, the teacher was not angry at him, and there were no fights with other children. But he was not ready to admit that it was difficult, or that it felt good to be behaving well, or in general, that he was behaving well. He just focused on his achievement: proving me wrong. I tried repeatedly to bring the issue back to how it was for him to feel that he had decided, he had invested effort, and he was successful in behaving better. It took about two sessions until he was ready to admit that, actually, he felt better when he behaved better. It took about two more weeks before Guy was able to accept my redefinition of his aggression as a behavior he himself was doing. I explained it as a way he thought would help him to control others. I also emphasized that it was up to him to change it, if he saw change to be important and was ready to invest the effort.

SCIM module 2: Problem analysis. I wanted Guy to learn about the cause–effect link existing between his behavior and the way others responded to him. Considering his staunch difficulty accepting responsibility for his own behavior, I thought it would be easier to start by observing others. Guy was asked to observe his classmates' behavior. First, I asked him to observe the way the teacher responded to various children in class. He could easily reply that the teacher did not respond uniformly. He was then asked to select two particular children for observation: one very good, quiet student and another child whose misbehavior exceeded Guy's. He returned with his conclusions: When the boy who was a good student answered the teacher's question, she smiled, and when he disturbed the teacher, she ignored it. However, when the "misbehaving" student failed to do his homework or talked aloud in the middle of class, the teacher became very angry. We analyzed these processes, focusing on the role of expectations and learning about the way in which a behavior occurs. Guy was soon able to comment that when a good student forgets to do homework, no one cares, but when a bad student forgets, the teacher gets angry. At first he criticized, "It's not fair. There's no justice in the world." But then he admitted that it is reasonable for the teacher to react that way, and he could understand it.

I asked him next to try observing his own behavior when he refrained from hitting, and to check if his emotions were different when acting in this new way.

Talking about cause and effect enabled me to start talking about the link between thoughts, emotions, and behaviors, and the way he could learn to control his thoughts. I started by presenting some exercises in the room. For example, in one exercise, I pushed Guy's hand and observed his response. I then asked him to explain why he was looking at me in such a strange, distant way. He answered: "Because you're really strange!" I encouraged Guy to think of additional possible interpretations for my action, and together we produced a list. We then went on to conjecture about Guy's ensuing feelings and behaviors, depending on the different thoughts he had about the reasons behind my action (see Table 11.1).

Table 11.1. List of Guy's Thoughts, Emotions, and Behaviors Regarding Tammie's Action

Event	Interpretation (thought)	Emotion	Behavior
Tammie pushed my hand	She hates me	Angry	Want to push her back
	She is strange	Surprised	Avoid touching
	She did it by mistake	Forgive her	Smile at her
	She wants to be friendly	Happy	Try to be friendly

To help Guy learn to identify the link between his own thoughts, emotions, and behaviors outside therapy, he was asked to keep a daily record of one event that occurred, noting his thoughts at the time, what kinds of emotions they aroused, and how he acted. At first, this assignment was difficult for him, so we practiced it as an imagery exercise. I invited him to close his eyes and try viewing himself playing in the schoolyard with his friends. He complied, and I asked him to look around at the other kids and see them. I then suggested that he try to focus more, and to see the way they were looking at him. Suddenly Guy shouted: "There's that bastard! He's laughing at me again! I'll show him!" He opened his eyes, and I asked him to describe what he had visualized. He told me about a child in the class who usually mocked at him. Guy said that the boy "was doing it again." I asked him to describe in detail the way this child looked, what he did, and how he behaved. It immediately became apparent that Guy was very impulsive in interpreting others' behaviors, tending to decipher every look as personally related to him and, usually, in a negative way. For the remainder of the session, I tried to encourage Guy to think about other alternatives that might explain that boy's smiling facial expression. It took a long while until Guy was able to give a neutral explanation like "maybe he's happy" or "maybe he heard a joke," rather than negatively ascribing the smile to himself.

For the next week, Guy was instructed to practice eliciting alternative interpretations for others' behaviors and to try to change his automatic, negative thoughts to positive, mediated ones. He had to repeat the same exercise we did together in the session, but this time, relating to his friends, and thinking for himself about the various alternatives. Finally, several weeks later, he was able to complete these tasks, but he continued to tell me that he was doing this only because I asked him to, and that actually he did not believe the other interpretations he had generated were true. I settled for this situation, for the time being; that is, it was unimportant whether or not he believed these alternative interpretations at this point, as long as he was capable of finding more positive interpretations for others' behavior. However, witnessing how entrenched Guy's negative emotions and perceptions were, I understood the need to work extensively in this regard.

SCIM module 3: Attentional focus. In this module, I thought Guy would benefit from learning to identify and discriminate his internal sensations and emotions, with an emphasis on Guy's focusing in on his feelings and predicting his own behavior. I asked him to try to monitor himself and listen for the very first internal cues that might tell him he was about to break down, shout, and explode. He was unable to complete this task, claiming that no such cues existed. So, once again, we practiced the task via an imagery exercise. This time, I asked him to close his eyes, take a deep breath, and focus on his own feeling. Then I suggested that he try to remember the big fight he had last week at school and to identify what he had felt then. He said he did not feel anything, but I saw him making fists with his hands. I asked him about that, and he opened his eyes and looked at his fists. He smiled and said he had never noticed that before. However, as we continued talking about the fight, Guy said that he thought he felt tension in his legs and hands before starting to argue. We tried other imagery exercises, where he had to view himself taking part in different arguments. Guy made fists during all those imagery exercises.

I asked him to record the feeling in his hands and legs every day for the next week. At the following session, Guy reported that he really was feeling tension in his muscles most of the time. I had also asked him to take the time to stand in front of a mirror and look at himself while angry. He reported that he thought he looked very red in the mirror when he felt enraged.

I discussed these physical phenomena with his parents, who corroborated Guy's fist making and red skin tone. I enlisted the parents' assistance, asking them to look out for these symptoms and to help Guy identify as soon as possible those times when he began to make fists or turn red. At that point, I did not want the parents to be more involved, because I was afraid it might provoke Guy's anger and rejection. Guy asked me to also notify his teacher and to request that she let him leave the classroom whenever she observed such a change in his face. I gladly assented. Later on, as Guy practiced self-control exercises, he learned to use relaxation, deep breathing, self-talk, etc. to calm himself.

To provide Guy with some tools for coping with these newly identified pre-outburst symptoms, we practiced deep relaxation exercises. At first, we focused mainly on helping Guy relax his hands and fists. He was instructed to practice the exercises daily. It was initially difficult for Guy to sit down, concentrate on those exercises, and practice them for the 15 minutes I assigned, so I asked him to do only part of the exercises. Slowly, Guy was increasingly able to use relaxation techniques to reduce his physical manifestations of rage, and he reported that thereby the internal feeling of anger was lessened at those times.

Gradually, Guy began to identify some of his emotions, referring to times he was very angry or furious, to times he was upset, and to times when he "felt nothing." I thought this was a good moment to start working on positive emotions as well. Guy was instructed to find something every day that made him feel good. It could be music, a talk with a friend, reading a book, etc. He was advised to write down one thing he did for himself every day, and to report how much he enjoyed it on a scale of 1–10. It was important for me to deal with imparting joy and happiness as well as reducing his aggressive behavior. I thought that Guy and his family were preoccupied by all his disruptive behaviors, and he had stopped becoming involved in positive activities that could make him happy. I thought it was time to move attention away from the problems, and focus more on positive feelings and behaviors.

SCIM module 4: Self-control exercises. In this last module, together, we pinpointed methods that could help Guy overcome his urge to impulsively hit someone. Guy had told me at one point that he wanted to be a television movie editor;

therefore, I utilized this personal area of interest by suggesting that he write a movie scene. He was very enthusiastic. I asked him to write a script about an aggressive boy. He was also given instructions on how to direct this scene. His task was to write instructions for the background music, sets, props, costumes, and actors' behavior. He created several scenes, eagerly going beyond the assignment. One of the most exciting scenes, reflecting his improvement, was a scene in a public playground. A seated boy was looking around while three children played football close by. The football hit the seated boy, and he just picked it up and threw it back to the group of children. Then the children started laughing at the boy, but he just turned, looked at them, smiled back, and picked up a magazine he was reading, ignoring them. At this time we had been discussing the strategy of ignoring others' disruptions, as well as using imagery methods to "keep his cool." In another scene, he described a boy starting to go toward a group of children to fight with them, as a little angel stood on his right shoulder smiling at him and showing him the car with the remote control that he wanted his parents to buy him. Immediately, the boy turned around and left those children alone. Guy was very proud of his scene writing, enjoying both the creative outlet and the sense of control it offered him over his characters. He was able to see tangible proof of his progress.

Within this fourth module, Guy also learned about the role of imagination, self-talk, reinforcement, and self-evaluation in controlling his behavior, and he began practicing these techniques. His instructions were to select one technique each day and then to try, first, to visualize himself practicing the technique and, second, to write down how realistic it seemed to him. Next, he had to attempt to apply the technique in real life. For example, when he selected the self-talk technique, Guy was taught to imagine he was very angry and then to try using self-instruction to calm himself down. During this exercise, he said things such as: "You're strong, you can control yourself!" or "It's better for you to stop now before you get punished" or "Mom will be proud of you if you succeed." In evaluating how realistic such self-talk appeared to him, to my great surprise, Guy assessed the last option (my mother will be proud of me) as a real possibility.

Phase 5 of Decision Making: Evaluating Guy at the End of Therapy and Maintaining Treatment Outcomes

Evaluation. About 3 months after we started therapy, a great decrease was evident in the frequency and intensity of Guy's aggression. However, only after eight months could I say that Guy had learned to control himself, increase his happiness, improve his social relationships, and learn to resolve his behavior problem. As we neared termination of therapy, it was time to evaluate Guy's progress.

Three techniques had helped me assess Guy in the beginning of intervention. I interviewed his teacher and parents and administered Achenbach and

Edelbrock's (1983) Child Behavior Checklist to each, and I interviewed Guy. Before ending treatment, I repeated those interviews and questionnaires. In line with the treatment goal of decreasing Guy's disruptive, aggressive behavior (see Table 4.8), these evaluation methods tapped his behavior change and focused on reports from the environment regarding Guy's functioning.

Both the parents' and the teacher's questionnaires revealed a remarkable change. Guy could no longer be assessed as aggressive. According to the questionnaires, he was considered a regular, normal boy.

In her interview, the teacher also reported striking improvement. She said Guy was not aggressive, got along very well with friends, and had returned to being a good student again. She reported that she herself had become very sensitive to his behavior. She said there were some days when he was not calm, and she saw him moving restlessly in his chair. On such days, she gave him special assignments, sent him out to relax, or made him sit next to her, and usually those solutions helped.

The parents said their son was much easier to handle, and they were very happy that there were no complaints from school. Although he remained cynical in his demeanor, this could now be seen as a sarcastic sense of humor rather than an angry attitude. However, they were still bothered by Guy's incessant quarreling with his siblings. Yet, they said that perhaps this was normal behavior in most families.

Guy himself declared that the greatest notable change had occurred in his teacher's and parents' behavior, because they had learned not to pressure him so much. Nevertheless, in this evaluative interview, when we started examining the way he responded now to social situations, Guy admitted that he had a much more positive attitude toward the world. He also pronounced "In the past, anyone could light me like a match, but now I'm the only one who can set the fire." Guy's own reports on his social relations and emotions provided crucial information in evaluating treatment outcomes, in line with the goal of increasing Guy's prosocial behavior and positive emotions (see Table 4.8).

Maintenance. As we entered the follow-up stage of intervention, I invited Guy to call me whenever he wanted to consult me or share something with me. I wanted to make sure he maintained the skills he gained, and that he continued practicing those skills (see Table 4.9). With adolescents, depending on how much change has become habitual, I generally suggest that phone calls be voluntary. Many teenagers, in the midst of a search for autonomy, prefer to cut off all contact with the therapist immediately. Guy called me twice in the first 3 weeks. Then, I did not hear from him for the next 3 months. As the school term ended, he came to me to show off his grades, happy to show me that he had received very good feedback in school. I have not seen him since.

An important feature of maintenance for Guy comprised the continuing support and reinforcement he received from his teacher. With the parents' consent,

I continued supervising the teacher for a few months after terminating Guy's individual treatment. She was a primary change agent during his therapy and became a primary maintenance agent, as Guy encountered new demands and challenges in school. Likewise, the parents' modified behavior continued to serve as a reinforcement of Guy's learned self-control skills at home.

12

Childhood Depression

LITERATURE REVIEW

The study of childhood depression has become increasingly popular in recent years, with particular focus on correlates of assessment and diagnostic criteria and on the relationship between depression in parents and their children (Kaslow et al., 1988). Studies have attempted to uncover the link between children's depression and a history of disturbances among parents. Biederman et al. (2001) recently found that parental major depression was associated with increased risks for social phobia, major depression, disruptive behavior, and poor social functioning.

For many years, the question has been debated as to whether children genuinely suffer from depression or whether they only exhibit transient moodiness that can be remedied with some well liked toy, candy, or other reward. The latter common attitude has been supported by psychodynamic approaches that view depression as a superego conflict that arouses guilt. Because the child's superego is not fully developed, clinical depression cannot exist (Beres, 1966). According to ego-analytic models of depression, depressed children's cognitive distortions are a function of problematic parent–child interactions that impair self-esteem, a perceived lack of instrumentality regarding the environment, and a dependence on significant others for gratification. These children's perceptions of their environment frequently render them unhappy (Bemporad, 1978).

Another approach to childhood depression is a view of the disorder as "masked." This position suggests that depression does exist in childhood, in the sense of an internal, unobservable pathological entity, the external manifestations of which are depressive equivalents. Children may be depressed, but this masked depression is manifested as a variety of behavioral complaints (Cytryn & McKnew, 1974). Masked depression is posited to include diverse disturbances such as enuresis, temper tantrums, hyperactivity, and so on.

A recent trend conceives depression as a comorbidity of psychiatric problems, linking depression with anxiety. Wadsworth and collegues (2001) suggested that the comorbid conditions of anxiety and depression, as assessed by the Child Behavior Checklist, can be considered as part of the same continuum of problems. Contrary outcomes were shown by Maubach (2000), who did not find evidence to support the hypothesis of a relationship between anxiety and depression.

Lefkowitz and Burton (1978) viewed depression as a transitory disorder. They emphasized that the symptoms are prevalent in normal children, disappearing over time and usually without clinical intervention, but remitting spontaneously.

Over the last decade, a consensus has emerged proposing that depression in childhood should be considered as similar to depression in adults (Kaslow et al., 1988). The main elements characterizing adult depression have also been found in children (Beck, 1963). The affective component characterizes both children and adults, encompassing dysphoria, mood change, weepiness, loneliness, and apathy. The cognitive component is similar at both ages as well, including low self-esteem, self-depreciation, guilt, indecision, and pessimism. The motivational component likewise typifies children, consisting of avoidance, escape, passivity, anergia, and decreased socialization. The psychomotoric components, such as sleep disturbance, appetite disturbance, and somatic complaints, are also evident in adults and children alike.

A review of the literature reveals that school aged children and adolescents experience not only the symptoms of depression, but also the depressive syndrome that impairs the child's functioning and includes a characteristic symptom pattern and duration (Kovacs, 1989).

Several features are crucial in order to define a child's disorder as depression: the persistence of the disorder for longer than two weeks, and at least four of the following symptoms: significant weight loss or weight gain while not dieting, sleep disturbance, psychomotor agitation or retardation, fatigue or loss of energy, feelings of worthlessness, diminished ability to think, recurrent thoughts of death, or suicidal ideation (*DSM-IV*, American Psychiatric Association, 1994).

In summarizing studies on depression, Kazdin (1988a) concluded that the area of assessment was underdeveloped. However, in the two ensuing decades, there has been much progress, and several assessment methods and self-report interviews have been developed for childhood depression.

Treatment

The most significant progress in the area of treating childhood depression is linked to the use of antidepressant medications for children (Kaslow et al., 1988). However, the effects of antidepressants are not yet clear, and studies reveal inconsistent outcomes. In a double blind, placebo-controlled study of major depression in childhood and adolescence, results showed that tricyclic antidepressants were not found to be effective (Ambrosini, 2000). In contrast, Waslick et al. (1999) reported good outcomes for antidepressant usage in chronic cases of depression. Significant drug effects emerged especially for the use of fluoxeteine and paroxetine.

Three major approaches to the treatment of childhood depression may be identified: pscychoanalytic, behavioral, and cognitive.

With regard to psychotherapy, psychoanalytic models for childhood depression focus on intrapsychic influences. Following Freud's (1957) theory, the psychoanalytic view of depression emphasizes the unsatisfied libidinal striving (usually parents who fail to fulfill the child's need) (Beres, 1966). The model focuses on the child's identification with the parent's values and ideals as playing an important role in the development of depression, as well as the evolution of self-criticism and self-rejection, which reflect anger and hostility. In the therapeutic process, depressed children learn to accept and be aware of their feelings toward the parents, to live with their anger and hostility, and then to replace the depression with more adaptive behavior.

The behavioral model for depression emphasizes environmental consequences as well as skills acquisition and deficits (Kazdin, 1988b). Most behavioral treatment models do not treat depression holistically. Rather, they focus on specific training in the particular domain in which the child suffers. Social skills training is one specific component that has commonly been included in depression therapy, in order to stop avoiding social activities and to obtain reinforcement from the social environment. Programs that increase activity level reflect the behavioral conceptualization of depression as reduced activity caused by a low rate of environmental activity. In addition, a prevalent treatment component comprises attribution retraining, which is based on the idea of learned helplessness. Attribution style filters experiences in such a way as to produce the deficits in affectivity, motivation, and self-esteem associated with depression (Kaslow et al., 1988; Kazdin, 1988b).

Cognitive therapy offers the depressed child a set of cognitive and behavioral strategies to help the child identify, reality test, and modify distorted conceptualizations and dysfunctional attitudes and beliefs. Cognitive techniques include: recognizing the connection between cognitions, affects, and behaviors; monitoring negative automatic thoughts; examining evidence for and against distorted automatic thoughts; substituting more reality oriented interpretations for distorted cognitions; and learning to identify and modify dysfunctional beliefs (Kaslow et al., 1988). Depression is emphasized as a deficit in interpersonal problem solving skills, highlighting the need to foster children's acquisition of those skills via treatment (Kazdin, 1988b).

The first stage in treating childhood depression consists of assessing whether the disorder is an outcome of another major childhood disorder that needs to be treated. In that case, treatment should first be aimed at alleviating these problems.

During the last decade, the focus of attention has shifted to treatment programs targeting the prevention of depression. Hannan and colleagues (2000) conducted a brief intervention program aiming to teach high school students in depression management strategies and positive coping skills. The results lent support to the effectiveness of this brief program for early intervention in childhood and adolescent depression.

Empirical reports on treatment of depression in children have been relatively sparse. The few case studies that have appeared revealed many methodological problems. Kazdin (1988b) concluded that much remains to be done in the domain of children's affective disorders. Some progress, especially in the development of assessment measures, can be noted in the decades subsequent to his study; however, the need still exists to identify developmental differences unique to the childhood disorders and to determine how best to address these peculiarities in treatment.

For instance, in trying to adapt Beck's (Beck et al., 1979) model of depression to children, I believe that several guidelines should be emphasized:

1. First of all, the need to establish an effective therapeutic alliance with the child, combining verbal and nonverbal communication.
2. The importance of involving the child's family in the treatment process.
3. The consideration of the child's cognitive development level, in making a decision regarding the central features of depression that should be addressed in treatment (e.g. guilt, self-concept, low self-criticism, etc.).

The following case study presents cognitive–behavioral therapy with an adolescent suffering from depression, integrating constructivist elements. I will try to address the developmental components, as well as the unique nature of childhood, to efficiently treat childhood depression.

JACOB: TREATING DEPRESSION AND HELPLESSNESS

I first saw Jacob two years before the therapy I will be presenting in this chapter. His parents came then to consult with me. Jacob was 15 years of age, at that time, and suffering from mild depression. He was using medications prescribed by a psychiatrist and in separate psychodynamic therapy. The parents said that a recent psychiatric assessment had revealed that Jacob was in danger of committing suicide, and the psychiatrist had wanted to hospitalize him. The parents had refused and decided to watch him carefully at home. They had come to my clinic, then, because Jacob's therapist was on vacation for two months, and the parents were very concerned about their son. They asked me to see him until his therapist returned.

At that interval, I met with Jacob about six times. He began to feel much better and wanted to continue treatment with me; however, I did not want to take him from his therapist, and I sent Jacob back to him. I spoke with the therapist and updated him on Jacob's condition. The therapist was very angry with me for initiating cognitive therapy in a severe depressive case, telling me I was treating the symptom instead of the real cause, and it was too dangerous.

Over the subsequent two years, I occasionally received telephone calls from Jacob's parents, telling me that nothing had changed dramatically and that they preferred returning to me. Finally, after two years, I agreed, on the condition that they discuss this with Jacob's therapist, tell him that they had not seen any significant results and had decided to return to me, and receive his agreement. When Jacob returned to my clinic, he was 17-years-old.

Preliminary Details: Assessing Jacob and His Family

Assessment of depression usually centers on interviewing the child directly and/or administering standard questionnaires for assessing depression (see increasing behavior in Table 4.2). The child is the most reliable source of information for overcontrolled, acting-in disorders. In Jacob's case, I did not administer standard tools because he had undergone all kinds of psychological and personality testing by his previous therapist, and Jacob felt these were useless. He did not want to complete any more questionnaires, and I decided to respect his wishes. I did not ask his previous therapist for written reports. There were two reasons for that. One, the therapist was very angry with Jacob and with me, and I did not want to turn to him and ask for such reports. Second, in a telephone call, the therapist shared his diagnosis and the outcome of different tests with me. It was all very psychodynamic, full of interpretations but with very little evidence, and I agreed neither with the diagnosis nor the view of therapy. I decided that I would rather look at Jacob from a new perspective and judge him in light of my view. I did, however, contact Jacob's psychiatrist, and decided to have consultation phone calls every few weeks.

In terms of Jacob's age, as an adolescent, he was certainly capable of reporting his own problems (see Table 4.3). Although parents are not a reliable source of information about their child's internal, affective disturbance, the family can be interviewed to provide additional particulars. I decided to first assess Jacob through a family interview, conducted to gather information about the whole family, and then to interview Jacob directly.

I met Jacob with his two parents. Jacob was the youngest child in the family. He had a brother aged 21 and a sister aged 24, both living at home. Both were very clever and successful. Both siblings had held very high positions in their mandatory military service and then became excellent university students. Jacob had very good relationships with them, especially with his brother, who was

Jacob's role model. Jacob came from a low middle class family. The father was a technician, and the mother was a secretary. Both of them were very protective, warm parents, who wished more than anything for their son to feel good. He had a very special relationship with his paternal grandparents and would spend a great deal of time with them. The mother's grandmother had suffered from depression and had received medication. She tried to commit suicide several times but died naturally of old age. Part of the parents' worries concerned their fear that Jacob had inherited his great-grandmother's depression.

The parents were very frightened. Even as we started therapy, and I knew they trusted me, they continued to take Jacob to undergo all kinds of assessments. They took him for psychological testing (to which I objected), then they went to a graphologist who said Jacob had some early severe trauma he was not revealing. They visited a fortuneteller, who told them that a bad spirit had entered their son's body and warned them to send bottles filled with prayers out to sea in order to save him. They went to an alternative treatment center, where Jacob received all kinds of herbs to drink. Although I talked with the parents often, I could not stop them from constantly looking for a cure. I understood their fears but felt they were not helping their son by dragging him around the city for help. Finally, I succeeded in at least gaining their agreement to go consult the various advice givers alone, without Jacob, and that they would not give him any medications without consulting me. From then on, they continued their pursuit of a cure by going to a rabbi, to a dream teller, and others, but without Jacob's knowledge.

Jacob was in the eleventh grade. He was studying in a multimedia education program in his high school and specializing in sound. He was usually an average student, but had shown some academic difficulties lately. He had many friends and good relationships with his peers, although gradually over the last two years he had seen them less and less often.

At the time of referral, Jacob was on antidepressant medication (Prozac) for his depression. Later on, during therapy, I consulted his psychiatrist, and we started gradually reducing the medication, until, by the end of treatment, he was able to stop it completely.

Assessing Jacob

The first part of this book mentioned direct observation as one of the most important methods for assessing children and adolescents. While trying to assess Jacob, the most meaningful data I obtained about his condition derived from looking at him, listening to him, and watching his behavior in our individual session. One of the most difficult tasks was conducting a full session with Jacob. He could not finish a sentence. He would start talking, use many words, apologize a lot, speak very quickly, and use considerable associative thinking. His sentences were very logical; however, they were so long and complicated, with so many question marks and emotions, that they were difficult to follow. He sounded so disorganized in the beginning that I wondered if he was losing touch with reality, and maybe developing a psychosis. Later on, I understood that Jacob was in touch with reality, but his pain and depression induced confusion and disorganization. The way he talked was the first sign that he was suffering from a comorbidity of depression and anxiety. His rapid, disorganized speech was much more typical of an anxiety disorder.

It was clear that Jacob was suffering. Mainly, he complained about feeling bad, lacking energy to do things, feeling the world was too complicated for him to cope with, feeling worthless and hopeless, and lacking the skills to cope with everyday tasks. When asked what exactly he felt, Jacob could not answer. His words were very generalized, holistic, and associative, like:

> Well, you know, I don't know, it's, like, you know, something, how can I say it? You know, I can't cope with, like, something, I don't know, I feel like I'm not doing things right. I want to, you know, but it's, like, I don't know, in a way, like, you know, everything is heavy, you know? I think things aren't, you know, the way they should be, I wonder, like, why I feel that way, you know...

As he spoke, Jacob would sit bending forward, with his head bent toward the floor and his hands moving constantly.

To try to cut through his nonstop talk, I decided to use imagery exercises (as I would extensively in future work with him). I asked him to describe himself using different metaphors. If he were a tree, what kind of tree would he be? He answered: "I would be a tree in the autumn, when all the leaves fall." As an animal, he described himself as a frightened rabbit. As weather, he said, "gray and cloudy," and as a color he chose black.

When I asked Jacob to describe his future, he replied, "If it continues like this, I don't know, I can't, it isn't possible. I won't make it, you know." I asked him if he really thought he was in danger of committing suicide, and he replied: "No, I couldn't do that to my grandparents. It would kill them. They're so good, you know, they don't deserve, like, you know, for me to do, you know... no, I don't think I would, but I wish it could happen, like, naturally..."

I asked him how he managed at school, and Jacob told me he was skipping school very often, did not take all his examinations, and stayed in bed a lot. He did not feel like meeting his friends, but he had one good friend who used to come to him, even if he did not want to see her. She was the one he was sharing all his thoughts and feelings with, and that helped a lot. He was eating very little and sleeping many hours, sometimes all day long. Lately, he even skipped some of the performances he used to take part in as a sound technician, and that got him into trouble with the orchestra he was working with.

Phase 1 of Decision Making: Does Jacob Need Therapy or Not?

In line with the different phases of decision making about therapeutic intervention presented in Chapter 4, the first decision concerned whether or not Jacob warranted treatment (see Table 4.1). In contemplating the problem variables, it was easy to assess Jacob as suffering from moderate depression disorder. He met all of the *DSM-IV* criteria (American Psychiatric Association, 1994). His disorder had been ongoing for more than two years and had affected all areas of his life: cognitive, emotional, social, and behavioral. Relating to cognitive distortions, Jacob presented low self-esteem, self-deprecation, difficulties in concentrating, and pessimism. He saw himself as worthless and as incapable of competing with his siblings. Jacob's affective disturbances included mood changes, weepiness, apathy, and anxiety. The fact that he also evidenced anxiety corresponds with the definition of childhood depression as incorporating a comorbidity of depression and anxiety (Wadsworth et al., 2001). Behaviorally, Jacob exhibited regressive behavior, lacked motivation or energy, and also presented psychomotoric depressive components such as sleep disturbances, appetite disturbances, and somatic complaints. With respect to his social relations, he had friends, but withdrew from social activities and would not initiate any meetings, so he met friends only once they called him or came to visit him. As for school, he was often truant, staying in bed instead. He missed lessons, did not do his homework, and avoided taking tests.

I did not see him as in danger in terms of suicidal ideation, and I sent him for a psychiatric consultation, which corroborated my evaluation. However, I thought Jacob showed deep problems that needed to be resolved, and I could easily assess his behavior as depression. I also saw signs of anxiety. It was not social anxiety, because he was not afraid of going out, but he was afraid of not being accepted and not being appreciated, and he worried a great deal about what others thought of him.

In relation to the frequency of the problem, it did not change over the prior year, and its severity did not lessen, but rather worsened. As for the question of future risk, as an adolescent, Jacob needed to be involved in peer relationships. Social activity was important for his well-being and identity formation, and the lack of this activity could harm his development.

The second variable in deciding whether or not to treat Jacob concerned developmental components. Jacob's functioning obviously differed from that of his age, sex, and cultural groups. His depression was much more severe than the usual moodiness or affective fluctuations characterizing this age.

In terms of child and family variables, the family was very motivated to help Jacob resolve his difficulties, and they were more than ready to cooperate with treatment assignments. Jacob, on the other hand, was not very highly motivated to change, but I interpreted this as rooting from his depression, rather than reflecting an objection to collaborating with therapy.

An examination of the treatment variables in Jacob's case suggested a high probability that he could be helped. Although depressed, he was still functioning in some areas of his life. He was avoiding social activities, but had good friends who cared for him and still kept in touch. He had started missing school, but was still a good student and cared about his grades. Mostly, he loved and cared for his family and was ready to do things for them. These attitudes implied that Jacob would also be likely to create a therapeutic alliance with me. It seemed as if this was a mild to moderate rather than severe depression, and still in a stage when prognosis was good, especially in light of Jacob's very good support system in the form of friends, teachers, and family. I therefore believed there was a promising chance to elicit change in this young man. The first phase of decision making highlighted the importance of treating Jacob's depression and anxiety.

Phase 2 of Decision Making: Classifying Jacob's Referral and Goals for Change

Now, the second phase was directed toward assessing the referred disorder in light of the four goals of childhood therapy (decreasing a behavior, increasing a behavior, removing anxiety, and facilitating development), and the relevant developmental tasks. Jacob could be evaluated as in need of two out of the four targets for changes (see Table 4.2): increasing his self-confidence and self-esteem, as well as eliminating his anxiety disorder. Both depression and anxiety can be classified as internal, acting-in disorders that characterize overcontrolled children. These disorders cause avoidance and regressive behavior. It was difficult to differentiate between the avoidance behavior caused by Jacob's depression and lack of energy, as compared to the behavior elicited by his anxiety, lack of confidence, and fear to fail. I therefore decided to design a treatment that would consolidate teaching Jacob how to give up his overly rigid control and how to expose himself to feared events (treating anxiety) with instructing him in how to increase his social and occupational activity and his self-awareness (treating depression). These goals correspond with the literature on the comorbidity of anxiety and depression among children and adolescents.

Looking at Jacob's developmental tasks (see Table 4.3), the adolescent stage requires developing self-identity and individualization from the family. Jacob exhibited problems in both areas. His poor self-esteem and self-confidence hindered his development as a self-assured adolescent. His feelings of inferiority and constant need to satisfy his parents' and grandparents' wishes impaired Jacob's ability to separate from his family and move soundly toward interpersonal peer relations and independent functioning. Both of these psychosocial developmental tasks should be addressed in therapy.

Phase 3 of Decision Making: Selecting Who Should Be Treated

To determine the optimal therapeutic setting, developmental considerations apply (see Table 4.4). As an adolescent, individual therapy would best suit Jacob, especially in view of his problems separating from his family. Working with Jacob solely within family therapy would thwart his capacity to express genuine needs and emotions, in that he would be preoccupied with complying with their wishes and expectations. Nevertheless, occasional sessions with Jacob and his parents together could potentially help the parents allow their son more autonomy and strengthen Jacob's self-esteem and assertiveness in dealing with his parents. A consideration of the treatment setting in light of Jacob's specific disorder also pinpointed the same decision (see Table 4.5). Increasing behavior and removing anxiety are problems that call for individual therapy. Nevertheless, as with all children's therapy, the parents should be involved. I decided to invite Jacob's parents to participate in supervision or counseling, with an emphasis on helping them cope with their son's condition and encouraging them to let Jacob "grow up."

Phase 4 of Decision Making: Selecting Jacob's Optimal Treatment Modes

Based on age considerations, Jacob could enjoy verbal, direct therapy conducted to impart social skills, cognitive restructuring, and coping skill techniques (see Table 4.6). However, the internal affective nature of Jacob's disorder (depression and anxiety), necessitated experiential and practice techniques in addition to verbal therapy (see Table 4.7). Moreover, in light of Jacob's unclear, confused verbal communication, it would be very difficult to base therapy primarily on verbal interaction. To help Jacob overcome and change his behavior, it seemed that a combination of verbal therapy and experiential techniques was in order.

Treatment Contract

The treatment contract included Jacob and his parents. Jacob agreed to enter individual therapy with me, and the parents agreed to let Jacob be independent and not interfere with his therapy. However, Jacob was very happy to give me permission to occasionally see his parents for supervision sessions. We agreed that the supervision would help the parents stop looking at Jacob as a sick child who needed to be freed of all responsibility at home. Also, we decided to have a family session for Jacob and his parents once every several weeks, to address issues disturbing all of them.

Counseling and Supervising Jacob's Parents

The intervention with Jacob's parents included counseling and supervision for them, and family sessions that included Jacob and his siblings. During the year I treated Jacob, I met with his parents for supervision every 4–6 weeks.

The counseling sessions were devoted to two main issues. The first was to update and reassure Jacob's parents. I updated them on his condition, listened to their fears and anxieties, and tried to help them relax. The fact that Jacob's mother in particular was intent on continuing her quest for a cure, by consulting a long list of different kinds of helpers, clarified to me how important it was to talk with them and reassure them. Although Jacob seemed to be very depressed, I was aware of his resources. Unlike many other depressive children, he had not lost interest in what was going around him, and was ready to be involved and help when others were in trouble. He demonstrated strong loving emotions and cared about his parents and grandparents, which I saw as good signs that could help him recover.

The second aim was to guide them in how to relate to Jacob. Because of their fears, the parents were overly protective of Jacob. They thought that by preventing him from experiencing any stress, they might help him feel better. Therefore, they had asked the school to release him from some assignments. They permitted him to stay at home and not go to school, never asked him for any help around the house, and were afraid to show anger toward him when he did something against their wishes, such as coming home too late, skipping meals, and so on. I instructed them to start treating him the same way that they would treat any other normal child. I explained to them that he needed to be asked for help with the chores, and he needed discipline and limits. By excusing him from all responsibility, they were just promoting his conception about how sick he was.

Family Meetings

In occasional family meetings with Jacob and his parents together, we tried to construct new ways of talking and interacting in the family, changing the communication style and family roles. For example, Jacob looked up to his successful older brother and sister, and he felt certain that his parents were very disappointed by him, in comparison. He thought his siblings were smarter than he was, nicer than he was, altogether better than he was. In the family sessions, I encouraged Jacob to express this sense of inferiority to his parents, and then they were helped to talk about how proud they were of him, and how each of their children was different. It was true that his older brother excelled at computers, but Jacob was the most creative child in the family, and they enjoyed him for what he was.

In one of the family sessions, we addressed the issue of secrets in the family, which Jacob had mentioned in his individual session with me. I thought it was about time to openly discuss them in order for Jacob to feel better. I asked the parents to invite their other two children and the grandparents to the next session. In that crucially important extended family meeting, I helped Jacob tell his whole family what he felt like, being so overprotected and shielded by them, as if they did not really trust him, or expected something terrible to happen to him. I helped him ask them to let go of him, trust him, let him be independent, and not show their worries so much. As he spoke, he cried and apologized for making them sad, but they cheered him by noting how right he was, and that actually, he was grown up, they believed in him and trusted him to cope well.

I asked Jacob's mother and grandmother if he resembled his depressed great-grandmother. At first, the mother was angry with me for talking aloud about the "secret," but Jacob said he knew about it and knew he was having the same symptoms as his great-grandmother. His grandmother then pronounced that he was completely different from her. She told Jacob that her mother had been absolutely fine until the holocaust. Then, in that session, Jacob's 70-year-old grandmother related aloud to the whole family, for the first time, the story of her mother. Jacob's grandmother had immigrated with her parents to Israel in 1930 (at age 3), leaving their family behind in Poland. Shortly after the end of World War II, her mother went back to Poland to search for her parents and other family members in the aftermath of the holocaust. She stayed there for several months. Their town had been completely destroyed. She heard terrible stories about the deaths of her entire family. She returned to Israel but kept silent, trying to protect her family from learning of the atrocities that her parents had endured. During the next few years, the great-grandmother developed intense guilt feelings about leaving her parents behind in Poland (they had not wanted her to go), and she became depressed. She tried to commit suicide several times but did not succeed. As the grandmother finished her story, she turned to Jacob and said: "You see, she wasn't ill. She had reasons to feel what she felt. You are not like her at all, and this is not something that was passed down in our family genes." They all broke into tears, and Jacob asked if she would tell him more about the family when they got home. This session relieved Jacob's worries about inherited depression and also helped instruct the entire family in how to show Jacob more trust and less overprotection.

The family sessions were conducted throughout Jacob's whole treatment, contributing to his ability to change and overcome his difficulties.

Designing the Goals and Intervention Process with Jacob

In light of Jacob age's and the nature of his depressive and anxiety disorders, I decided to treat Jacob using mainly constructivist techniques while applying my SCIM training model, as described in Chapter 5. Self-control would assist Jacob to change his thinking style, set appropriate expectations and criteria for his behavior, develop awareness of his internal affective cues, and, most of all, cope with his inferior and despondent feelings. We were able to decide together on several main goals of our treatment. I thought Jacob was suffering from comorbid anxiety, depression, and low self-esteem. We needed to work toward multiple goals, but, first of all, I thought it was necessary to have him develop a daily routine. When he stayed home and stopped functioning, his situation deteriorated. I saw that he felt better when active, and I knew I could mobilize his motivation to design a daily schedule. The first goal, therefore, comprised increasing Jacob's activity and involvement in everyday tasks.

The second goal involved his anxiety. Jacob was afraid of not being accepted, not being good enough, and not succeeding in school the way he wished. I thought that working on decreasing his anxiety would facilitate his ability to be more involved in daily activity, which, in turn, would lead to a sense of competence and thus better moods. While the first two goals could best be achieved by application of cognitive techniques, the last two goals can best be achieved by using constructivist techniques.

The third goal targeted Jacob's thinking style. Jacob was characterized by negative cognitive patterns. He would think of himself as incompetent, and he believed others did not appreciate him and did not want to be with him. He needed to change his self-acceptance, self-confidence, and self-appreciation.

The fourth goal involved regular developmental issues impacting Jacob. As a 17-year-old, Jacob was exposed to a wide range of emotions and sensations with which he did not know how to cope. However, such emotions were a normal part of growing up in adolescence. I thought Jacob should learn more about what was normal for boys his age, to normalize and legitimize the feelings he had toward himself, his friends, and his family.

As a first step in empowering Jacob's self-esteem, I invited him to collaborate with me on making decisions about the goals of therapy. Not only did I want Jacob to take an active part in making decisions about the goals of therapy, but also, in view of his low self-confidence, I wanted to guide him in learning how to appropriately establish targets and expectations for his future. At first, true to his typical behavior when encountering something new, Jacob refused. Then, he said he did not know how. In discussing some possible treatment targets, I realized that Jacob was objecting to every attempt of mine to raise issues. Each made him feel anxious and uncertain. Also, verbal discussion was very difficult and tiresome. Since Jacob was a very creative boy, and his disorder was an emotional problem, the use of creative constructivist techniques seemed to be the treatment of choice. I therefore obtained his agreement to participate in some imagery and metaphor exercises that would help us decide on the treatment goals.

Employing Neimeyer's (1995b) method of laddering, I asked Jacob to imagine that there was a large ladder in the room. On the bottom rung, a sign read: "sorrow, fear, depression, and hopelessness." I asked him to imagine what would be written on the top rung, if it represented his full progress in therapy and if nothing stood in his way of changing himself in whatever direction he chose. I emphasized the fact that this was only imaginary, and that he could imagine whatever he liked when he pictured where he would like to be at the end of treatment, versus where he was now. On the top rung, he put: "happy, satisfied, feeling good with myself and others." It took him a long time to complete the other rungs, but eventually he offered the following ladder:

First rung:	Able to do ordinary things like to read, write, and talk with people
Second rung:	Able to concentrate on my studies
Third rung:	Improve my grades
Fourth rung:	Enjoy being with people
Fifth rung:	Feel hopeful, happy, and worthy, feel competent
Sixth rung:	Like my behavior and myself
Seventh rung:	Happy, content with myself and others

Utilizing this exercise helped us decide on Jacob's treatment goals:

To decrease depressive behavior
To increase his ability to function
To improve self-esteem
To learn to live with himself and others
To increase happiness and satisfaction

Starting to Treat Jacob

The first stage in treating Jacob, before starting our self-control training, targeted the first goal of intervention that I had devised, that is, to increase Jacob's activity and involvement in everyday tasks. I thought it crucial that Jacob develop regular patterns for eating, sleeping, and attending school. His parents' collaboration was enlisted to ensure that he would keep the new routine. Jacob was asked to attend school every day unless he was physically ill (fever, vomiting), and his parents were forbidden to let him stay home, even if he complained about feeling bad. He was instructed to report to me about his school attendance in daily telephone calls. Usually, when everything went well, he did not call me. His mother called me several times early in the morning, telling me Jacob would not wake up and refused to go to school. I asked to talk with him and persuaded him to go to school. At those times, he would call me in the evening to tell me he did go, and that it had been okay for him.

With regard to eating habits, Jacob was instructed to eat his meals with the family every day as they were accustomed, but without skipping any meals. He was told to go to sleep on time, and his mother was responsible for waking him up in the morning rather than letting him sleep, as before, for the whole day. At first, he complained, but soon he succeeded in adhering to the new routine and then felt better about his ability to function.

Also, I asked Jacob to keep a chart of the social activities in which his class was involved, and to try to become involved in as many as possible, even though he did not enjoy being with his peers. He was instructed to participate regularly in the local youth group and as editor of the school newspaper, two activities that had previously been sporadic. In addition, he was asked to record his leisure activities and bring the chart to the session, to ensure that he was meeting with his friends over the weekends.

As soon as Jacob started to become more active again, a remarkable improvement appeared in his depressed mood. He still complained about a lack of energy, depression, and difficulties in coping, but he was now attending school regularly and becoming involved in peer activities. In conjunction with his problems, Jacob could also report some joy and happy feelings. Now we could start working toward imparting self-control skills to Jacob.

SCIM module 1: Cognitive restructuring and redefinition. Jacob conceptualized himself as a sick teenager. He would say that he was a bona fide depressive personality, meaning that there was no reason to try and do things that had no chance of working. He was depressed and would always be depressed. This view of himself as a sick person caused Jacob to give up; he made no effort to change or to take on responsibility for change, but rather simply waited for his sickness to magically disappear. The more he looked at himself as sick, the sicker he felt and behaved. In this first training module, I aimed to help Jacob reconstruct the way he looked at himself, and to facilitate his understanding that he was responsible for his own behavior and feelings.

During the first month, Jacob insisted that he had many things to tell me and needed time. Throughout the whole session, he spoke rapidly in his disorganized manner and encountered many instances when I did not understand what he wanted to say, but he would not let me interfere. For the first four individual sessions, I sat quietly, letting him talk. I felt I needed to meet him on his ground, at his tempo and pace. So, I kept quiet, suggesting once in a while that we should try some exercises. He refused.

During the fifth session, he was complaining about how depressed he felt, and how helpless he was. I said that that was what he chose to feel. If he did not want to be depressed, he could start doing something to change it. He said he would if he knew how, and then I once again offered that he try doing some exercises with me. He agreed this time, and we began with guided imagery.

I thought that imagery exercises might assist Jacob in relinquishing control and in giving up his need for analytic thinking, thereby enabling him to act differently. I asked Jacob to relax and then to imagine he were sitting in front of a video screen. I asked him to imagine that he was watching a movie of himself on the video screen, and I wanted him to concentrate on how he looked, what he was doing, and how he sounded. I emphasized that he should observe his own gestures, tones of voice, and word choice.

We focused on the details of this picture for about half of the session. Jacob acknowledged that he did not like what he saw. He was speaking too fast, was too nervous, had a high voice, and his words were unclear and confused. There was a lot that he wanted to change. After some time looking at himself this way, he was ready to admit that he had not always been this way, he used to be different.

I asked him to try and bring up the picture of himself before he became depressed. As he did, Jacob began to cry, telling me that he used to be a nice, happy, social boy. I asked him to try and concentrate on this happy picture during the following week, and to try pinpointing the differences between himself in the present and himself in the past. Then, we could use those differences as goals to work toward.

Toward the end of this session, Jacob asked me several times if I believed he could be what he was before. Each time, I answered that no one can return to what they were before, because we all keep changing and growing, but that I was sure he could change and improve if he worked on it.

In the next session, I introduced Mahoney's (1991) stream of consciousness method. Stream of consciousness invites clients to simply examine themselves and their lives *in vivo* in the session. In this exercise, the client is invited to attend to and, as best as one can, report ongoing thoughts, sensations, images, and feelings. This technique falls into the flexible focus (mindful) class of meditative exercise. The person's privacy needs are honored in stream of consciousness reporting. Therapist interpretations are not considered the primary or ultimate authority on their meaning (Mahoney, 1983), and clients are asked to encourage and respect the ebb and flow in their ability and willingness to share the content of the immediate experience.

Once again, I asked Jacob to relax, this time lying down. Then I suggested that he concentrate on himself and talk associatively, without thinking, about anything and everything that came into his mind. As he started talking, I was very surprised to note that he spoke clearly and fluently, without hesitation, stops, or complex sentences. So, I asked him what would he like to change and do with himself. Jacob said that it was very important for him to be nice to people, help other people, interact with others, and feel appreciated by them.

When we were talking about this exercise, I asked Jacob if he thought he could talk the way he talked if he was really sick and if the depression was out of his control. Jacob was also surprised to hear to his own clear speech, and admitted that maybe he was capable of communicating differently. For the next few sessions, we focused on the different ways in which Jacob increased his own distress. For example, his negative self-talk, and the way he always thought he knew what others were thinking, and how he always interpreted it in a negative way. The way he compared himself with his siblings, feeling inferior, and his withdrawal from activity that caused him to stay at home and not enjoy life like others. Jacob started to voice the suspicion that perhaps his belief of himself as sick and helpless was untrue. He even stated: "Maybe, if I work hard, and if I knew how, I could make some changes." I felt we were progressing and could start working toward other goals.

Another imagery exercise that helped us reconstruct the way he thought of himself consisted of Wozner's (1985) "evaluation circle" technique. I told him: "Each of us has many circles of people we know. In each circle, people know us in a different way. The closer they are to us, the more they know about us. So, how about if we learn what you would see if you were other people looking at yourself? Let's start with strangers, people on the street, the farthest and most distant circle. If you walk in the street, and people you don't know see you, what would they see?" Jacob said that they would see a nice looking, young, shy boy walking around. Next, I asked him, "Now, imagine this time you're being watched by a kid from your class, someone who sees you every day. What would he think of this Jacob guy?" He smiled and answered that Jacob is a very friendly, nice, creative kid, and all the girls love him. We continued with the closer circle of his family, and eventually with what he saw when he looked at himself.

Later on, I asked Jacob why everyone sees him in such a nice way except himself. After thinking for a while, he replied: "Maybe that's because the problem is not what I am, but what I think of myself, and maybe others are right, but I don't really feel it." This was very important progress, and I realized that Jacob was beginning to recheck his own cognitions and search for other meanings in his behavior; that is, he was ready for the second module of the SCIM.

SCIM module 2. Problem analysis. At this stage in the intervention process, Jacob had to learn about the links between his thoughts, his emotions, and his behaviors, to identify the cause and effect process. I asked Jacob to record difficult events that occurred during the upcoming week, using a chart to try to link his thoughts and interpretations to his emotions and behaviors. In the next session, he showed me his chart. He had recorded many events, but had given them all self-deprecating interpretations that could be summed up as "I'm a failure" (see Table 12.1).

I asked him to try changing those interpretations. We worked on this together, and with my help he was able to elicit possible new interpretations (see Table 12.2). I checked with Jacob to see if these alternative options sounded right to him.

When Jacob was ready to accept these interpretations, we tried to see the difference in his emotions elicited by the new interpretations. Jacob practiced this exercise for 3 weeks before he was able to say that he could see how much his feeling could change, once he tried to alter the meaning he attributed to an event. For

Table 12.1. Jacob's First Chart of Events and Their Interpretations

Event	Interpretation
I invited a friend over, but he didn't come.	Kids don't like me.
A girl I like didn't smile at me in school.	She doesn't like me.
I received a B on a test.	I can't handle my studies.
My parents didn't let me go out.	They don't trust me.

Table 12.2. Jacob's Revised Chart of Events and Their Interpretations

Event	New interpretation
A friend didn't come over.	Maybe he was busy and couldn't come.
The girl didn't smile at me.	She was probably preoccupied by some problems of her own.
I received a B on the test.	I'm lucky I didn't fail, because I didn't prepare at all, and I was very depressed.
My parents didn't let me go out.	They're very worried about my condition and fear something might happen to me.

example, instead of thinking that his peers came over to visit because they felt sorry for him, he started telling himself that they came over because they liked him and enjoyed being with him. Instead of feeling insulted when a friend did not come, he would feel sorry that he had not had the chance to be with that friend.

SCIM module 3: Attentional focus. This module aimed at teaching Jacob to identify his internal cues. He tended to interpret each stimulus as distress or a sign of depression. He needed to learn to identify feelings of anxiety, excitement, and anger, rather than focusing only on sorrow. It was also important to teach him to differentiate between times he felt only a little depressed and times he felt very depressed, and to see the link between his internal cues and the emotions he reported.

These goals were achieved via relaxation and concentration exercises. Jacob was instructed to concentrate on the inside of his body and to identify his physical sensations, their location, and their intensity. Then he tried to see whether or not he could link the physical stimuli to emotional sensations. We practiced the exercise in the treatment sessions, and Jacob had to do the same at home. During the week between sessions, his assignment was to record:

What did I feel
Where exactly did I feel it
When did it happen
How strong was it

Next, he had to think whether there could be other interpretations for his sensations that differed from what he originally thought. After several practice sessions, Jacob was able to say: "I felt something strange in my throat. I used to think it was a sign of anxiety. Maybe it isn't. Maybe I just didn't drink enough." Or, he told me: "There's something in my stomach. I'm not sure if it's excitement or anxiety. I'm not sure." These reflected Jacob's attempts to start appropriately identifying his internal cues without relying on his automatic thoughts.

We conducted another imagery session targeting Jacob's ability to identify his internal stimuli. By that time, Jacob had already practiced many imagery exercises. Having studied art, and being as creative as he was, he had already started enjoying these exercises and gladly participated in them. This time, I asked Jacob to imagine he was a very small person, as small as his pinky finger. He then took a trip inside his own body. I asked him to enter his body and wander around. He was told to notice where he was, how he felt in each place, what it looked like from the inside, and what he saw. At first, the task was very easy for him. He walked around inside his legs, stomach, and hands and, with great humor, described his nice sensations and feelings. However, when he reached his throat, Jacob began saying how badly he felt. He said it was very narrow and there was pressure. He felt as if he was struggling, and almost could not breathe. When I asked what made it so unpleasant, he said: "the words that I dare not let out." We stopped the exercise at that point, and began discussing the meaning of his fear to talk. He talked about how important it was for him to please everyone, and how difficult it was to express negative emotions, especially toward those who cared about him. In the next module of self-control practicing, Jacob had to practice talking with others and expressing his wishes and thoughts with his parents, siblings, and grandparents.

In the next session, we returned to this inner body trip exercise. It was still difficult for him to enter his throat, but he was able to express some feelings while there. He then moved to his heart and said he was burning and could not stay there. As we discussed this, I realized that those feelings were age related. It was hard for Jacob to deal with the romantic feelings he had toward a girl in his class, he was afraid of love, and was afraid of hurting her. Again, as his depression decreased, we started focusing much more on his peer relationships and normal responses toward peers, and I helped Jacob deal with those emotions.

We therefore started working on the fourth module of imparting him with self-control skills to improve his coping with the difficulties he faced.

SCIM module 4: Self-control exercises. In this module, in order to promote his self-control skills, Jacob first practiced exposure therapy aiming to decrease anxiety. Jacob was given assignments that he had to complete daily. The tasks involved exposure to his feared situations – handing in class assignments, raising his hand in class, daring to invite a friend over, and so on. Jacob practiced this using three steps (Marks, 1969, 1978, 1987). First, he rated his anxiety before being exposed, on a scale of 0–10. Second, he had to decide he was going to stop his avoidance behavior, start doing something that was difficult for him to do, and thus become exposed to the feared event. Third, Jacob had to wait until the anxiety decreased and then rate the anxiety again, using self-talk to encourage himself and compliment himself for success.

Jacob succeeded in each assignment that he undertook, which enabled him to see that the fear stemmed from his own dread of failure rather than from realistically being unable to perform these tasks.

In his day-to day conversation, Jacob often used the metaphors of sinking and drowning. I decided to use client-generated metaphors to help him identify his feelings in his own words (Kopp, 1995). As Mahoney (1991) and Kopp (1995) noted, working with metaphors is not working word by word, proposition by proposition, testing each out against the current standards of evidence, but instead proceeds on a more holistic level whereby the adaptation of a new language game itself ushers in new standards. As mentioned before, client generated metaphors aim to enhance the therapist's understanding, feeling, and/or coping with a situation in therapy, and to facilitate the construction and design of the session. This technique is directed toward the feature of cognitive behavioral therapy related to goal-directed processes, as well as to practicing and experiencing processes. When the therapist deems a client proposed metaphor to be useful in progressing toward treatment goals, the therapist asks the client to fill in the lacking details (e.g. "What kind of equipment do you think you should carry with you on your trip?") (Kopp, 1995).

Jacob referred often to drowning; therefore, we used the metaphor of himself as someone sinking in the mud. I asked Jacob to look around himself while he was sinking, and to see what and who were there. He described many people around him trying to keep him from sinking, but no one succeeded. He felt he was sinking deeper and deeper. I asked him to describe what he felt, and he said: "It's mud. It's very heavy, I'm falling down, and there is the strong smell of mud with rotten leaves, and it stinks. It's dark, and it's getting harder to breathe." Then I asked him if there was anything good about it, and he said: "You know, I don't need to fight. I can just be there, because if I try to get out, I only sink deeper. It's a strange feeling just to be there, I don't need to do anything. I can rest. Well, if I don't die, if it's not the end, if it doesn't get into my mouth and nose, maybe I will even enjoy it."

Later on, I asked Jacob what it meant for him to be in the mud. Using a metaphor to explain another metaphor, he said that at first it was like knocking his head on a wall. I connected to this new metaphor and asked what it meant for him to stand near a big wall, knocking his head on it. He said it hurt, he was bleeding, and he did not like the idea. I asked if it lasted long. He replied: "No, suddenly it was pleasant. Not being hurt anymore, being relaxed. I asked what that meant for him, and he answered: "Maybe I started believing that someone would get me out. Yes, maybe I believe you'll get me out."

It was interesting the way his metaphors placed him in jeopardy but also tried to find ways for him to be rescued. I asked: "How could I help you?" and he suggested: "I think you could throw me a very long, strong rope. I can hold it tightly and try to pull myself out." He refused to answer what that rope might be, but I ended that session saying that, "Yes, I'll be happy to throw you a rope. All you need to decide is what's in that rope, how I can help you get out."

At the next session, Jacob came back, saying: "I guess you need to help me love myself and think that I'm good." This was about the end of the fourth month of intervention. Jacob was feeling much better. He was following my instructions and completing all his homework assignments, was attending school, and was participating in all his activities. He was much more organized and less confused, although he still suffered from mood changes and felt worthless.

I thought it was time to find out the causes and reasons for his feelings, and I proposed we draw a road map. The map reflected where he was at, his destination, and the road he wanted to take to get there. In order to drive well, with no accidents, and to arrive safely, we needed some warning signals.

The metaphor of life as a journey or a road allows for the consideration of difficulties, alternatives, and solutions. In the global constructivist therapeutic process called meaning making, the focus can alternately widen and narrow according to the client's need (Carlsen, 1995). Metaphors are meaning transports, which extend our level of understanding via a comparison, or some might argue by smuggling extra dimensions into our analysis (Olds, 1992). The metaphor of life as a journey suggests maps and turning points, landmarks, barriers and breakthroughs, steps and stages, high points and low, states of being lost and states of finding oneself (Carlsen, 1995). All these can help foster creativity in discovering new ways of coping.

We thus used this metaphor of a road. I asked Jacob to put signals and signs on his road map. He inserted several kinds. At one level, Jacob added actual traffic warning signs: dangerous curves, sharp detour, do not drive so fast, pay attention to pedestrians. Then he hesitated and added other, personal signs: be careful! successful brother; stay back! too much affection; go back! you might get burned by mother's love; hide! grandparents are too worried. The latter signals gave us insight into the problems caused by his so-called "good family relationships." They were too protective, permitting no expression of Jacob's genuine experiences in these relationships. He felt he could not compete with his siblings; his grandparents' overconcern annoyed him and made him feel guilty for not behaving the way they expected; and his mother's love was smothering him.

In the next session, we worked on guided imagery again. I asked Jacob to imagine there was a war going on in his mind between his depressed mood and his happiness. I asked him to visualize the battle and put words into each of the parties' mouths. At first, as speaker for the depressive moods, he declared: "I have to be depressed. The world is a bad place to be. Too many problems. Too many sorrows. People are hurt all the time. No one can be happy." But then, in the name of the happiness, he proclaimed: "Well, everyone has to do what they can. I have a family that many people don't. I'm loved. I'm healthy. I exist. Isn't that enough reason for happiness?" I asked him if he could permit himself to be happy, and we ended the session with him admitting there was nothing he wanted more than that.

The next few sessions were devoted to helping him accept himself more fully by pinpointing all his good characteristics, teaching him self-talk to flatter himself, and focusing on his good nature. We played the "supermarket game of characteristics," where each of us had to try to sell the other some unwanted characteristics of ourselves and to buy some good attributes from the other. As we played, he realized that there were many things he was not ready to give or sell me. He loved his ability to be sensitive and considerate of others, he loved his ability to think and imagine things, he loved his ability to enjoy music and intimate conversations with friends and to share feelings. Actually, the only things he wanted to change were his height (he felt he was too short), his moods, and the way he exaggerated and took things to the extreme. After this session, he stopped talking about himself as worthless and started thinking how he wanted to improve.

He asked me to teach him relaxation, and we practiced deep relaxation. I also taught him to use self-guided imagery to improve the way he felt about things. We attempted to determine which specific situations or people made him feel degraded or worthless, and he discovered that he was unable to: (1) cope with criticism without seeing it as the end of the world, (2) express negative emotions such as anger, and (3) assertively stand up for his way of dealing with things.

We devoted several sessions to assertiveness training, talking about the skills he needed to acquire and then role playing situations and rehearsing techniques. Finally, I asked Jacob to practice these assertiveness techniques by applying them in his natural environment, with his friends. It was not easy for Jacob to be able to say: "I'm sorry, but I can't prepare this activity for the youth group for tomorrow. I'm too busy. I have a test. It will have to wait until next week." However, slowly, he improved, and his parents admitted at that time: "He's not as easy and cooperative as he used to be. He's learned to say no, and we're not sure we like the idea..." Yet they laughed, commenting that they never thought he was paying such a high price for being so good, and all they ever wanted for him was to be healthy and enjoy life.

As Jacob practiced stream of consciousness again at this point, he sounded completely different. He talked slowly about the good things in his life. He spoke about his wish to have a girlfriend, his fear of whether he would be able to truly love her, and his fears about being able to have "normal and satisfying sex." These sounded very much like the problems typifying most adolescents his age. In light of the fact that Jacob was no longer depressed and had gained the necessary skills to cope with his daily problems, I was able to focus on verbal therapy for the next six weeks. Through conversation, we dealt with his social relationships, maturing identity, first love and affection, as well as sex and intimate relationships. After almost one year of treatment, it seemed termination was near, and evaluation was in order.

Phase 5 of Decision Making: Evaluating Jacob at the End of Therapy and Maintaining Treatment Outcomes

Evaluation. Assessment at baseline had focused on the parents' report and on Jacob's self-report and charts. In line with the recommendations outlined in

Table 4.8, the optimal evaluation methods comprised Jacob's reports of his social relations and emotions, as well as his parents' reports on his behavior. Thus, at the end of the treatment, we held another family meeting, where I asked everyone (parents, grandparents and siblings) for their feedback on Jacob's behavior, and I assessed Jacob individually.

At the family meeting, the parents as well as his siblings were very happy to tell me that Jacob was now acting like everyone else. He was happy again, doing well in school, was nice company at home, and they did not see any problem. The father smiled and said that he started rebelling several times, which he never dared do before. He said he was not happy when his son defied the father's wishes, but he also knew it was normal behavior for an adolescent.

In an assessment session with Jacob, I asked him to bring some of the audiotapes he had recorded at the beginning of our treatment. At that time, Jacob was afraid he would not remember what I said, because he was so depressed, so he used to tape all our sessions. I asked him to listen to those old tapes and look for the changes. Jacob was shocked to listen to himself. He said that everything had changed: his voice, the tempo of his speech, the volume, the content of the words.

Assessment of his current behavior revealed that Jacob was eating, sleeping, going to school, and studying. Also, his moods had changed, and he was no longer depressed. Moreover, he was happy and very much involved in peer activities. Evaluation enabled us to state that Jacob had very much progressed and now could no longer meet any clinical diagnostic criteria.

Maintenance. We terminated therapy after a year, with my promise to see him in the future whenever he felt the need to talk with me. At first, he returned for follow-up sessions every 4 weeks. After 3 months, he called me and said it was difficult for him to come. He was graduating high school at that time, and soon after, he was drafted into the army. He called me to let me know he was going into the army, and was happy that he could do his mandatory service as a sound technician in a military band. His mother called me twice to update me on how well he was doing, and I did not hear from them again.

IV

Summary and Closing Remarks

13

Linking the Theoretical Ground and Case Studies in Light of the Different Phases of Intervention

In the present book, I tried to familiarize the reader with the importance of flexible thinking that enables the integration of various components into one coherent entity, consisting of creatively implemented cognitive–constructivist therapy to address children's and adolescents' disorders. Three domains were targeted for integration: developmental and clinical concepts; cognitive and constructivist theoretical approaches; and goal-directed, designed therapy with a flexible, relationship-based approach.

First, I tried to integrate two different approaches to children's treatment. The first, the clinical approach, emphasizes assessment and intervention based on the clinical definition of childhood disorders and goals of treatment (*DSM-IV*, American Psychiatric Association, 1994). The second, the developmental approach, underscores normal developmental process as the basis for making decisions about children. The integration of these two approaches can be seen in Figure 13.1. The figure summarizes the different phases of intervention, first in light of the clinical division (problem types) and then in light of developmental components.

Second, I tried to integrate two ground theories: the cognitive and the constructivist. From the standpoint of both the cognitive and the constructivist theories, various disorders result from the specific human construction and organization that gives patterns and direction to one's life. The cognitive elements focus on identifying the link between thoughts, emotions, and behaviors (Beck, 1976). They also aim at changing automatic thoughts to mediated ones and at

	PHASE 1	PHASE 2	PHASE 3	PHASE 4
AIM	Decision on need of therapy	Classifying referral & goals	Selecting appropriate setting	Selecting treatment techniques
VARIABLES TO CONSIDER	1. *Problem variables* 2. *Developmental & environmental variables* 3. *Child & family variables* 4. *Treatment variables*	1. *Problem type:* Decreasing behavior Increasing behavior Removing anxiety Facilitating development 2. *Developmental stage:* Infancy Early childhood Middle childhood Adolescence	1. *Problem type:* Decreasing behavior Increasing behavior Removing anxiety Facilitating development 2. *Developmental stage:* Infancy Early childhood Middle childhood Adolescence	1. *Problem type:* Decreasing behavior Increasing behavior Removing anxiety Facilitating development 3. *Developmental stage:* Infancy Early childhood Middle childhood Adolescence
AVAILABLE DECISION	Must be treated Treatment recommended Doesn't need treatment	Determining the objectives and targets of intervention	Parents group Parents counseling Environment counseling Family therapy Individual therapy	Direct therapy Indirect therapy Verbal therapy Nonverbal therapy

Continued

	Treatment	PHASE 5
AIM	Implementing the self-control intervention model (SCIM)	Evaluating & maintaining outcomes
TECHNIQUES	1. *Cognitive restructuring* 2. *Problem analysis* 3. *Attentional focus* 4. *Applying self-control skills*	*Evaluation* Return to baseline assessment measures *Maintenance* Generalization & transfer Overlearning Relapse prevention Charting Practicing
AVAILABLE DECISION	Continual assessment to validate decisions made in Phases 1 through 4	*Evaluation* Were goals achieved? *Maintenance* Selecting appropriate tools for follow up

Figure 13.1 Summary of the Cognitive–Constructivist Process for Children and Adolescents

imparting clients with the necessary skills for overcoming problems (Ronen, 1997b). The constructivist elements, on the other hand, focus on promoting meaning making activity (Neimeyer, 1995b) and on helping clients explore possible avenues for movement while respecting the core organizing principles on which their views of life are built (Neimeyer, 1995a; Mahoney, 1991). The combination of cognitive and constructivist therapies fosters the integration of empirical assessment, decision making processes, techniques for helping clients overcome and cope, and evaluation and maintenance of treatment outcomes. The integration of the two approaches is conducive to the development and the application of more flexible methods. These methods target acceptance, change, and the identification and reformulation of central metaphors that inform the client's self-narratives. The blending of these two theories enables therapists to relate to and facilitate knowledge about human affective experience, in a manner that is infused with significance and can itself be viewed as a refined form of knowing (Neimeyer, 1995b).

As can be seen in Figure 13.1 (under the subheading of treatment), I have linked these two theories into one unified approach to analyzing and conceptualizing children's disorders and treatment. I proposed that cognitive–constructivist therapy for children be a goal-directed intervention aimed at teaching self-help skills to children and adolescents. For this purpose, I proposed the self-control intervention model (SCIM) that includes four modules: cognitive restructuring, problem analysis, attentional focus, and self-control training.

Third, I attempted in this book to integrate the importance of predesigned, goal-directed therapy, which is planned during an ongoing process of decision making about treatment, on the one hand, with an emphasis on flexible, creative techniques and therapeutic relationships as the major means to achieve change via the treatment process, on the other hand. The designed, goal-directed aspect of therapy can be seen in the decision making process illustrated in Figure 13.1, whereas the creative and relationship aspects of treatment will be elaborated in Chapter 14.

As can be seen in the figure (and as described in detail in Chapter 4), assessment constitutes a designed process of decision making relating to the child's characteristics, problems, development, and needed goals for intervention. As elaborated in Chapter 4, Phase 1 is directed toward determining whether or not the child necessitates treatment in light of problem variables, developmental variables, child and family variables, and treatment variables. Phase 2 of decision making is directed toward classifying the child's disorder in light of the kind of the problem (needing a decrease in behavior, an increase in behavior, the removal of anxiety, and/or the facilitation of development). Also, this phase is directed toward developmental stages: infancy, early childhood, middle childhood, and adolescence. During Phase 3, the appropriate setting(s) are selected for assessment and intervention. The available settings include parent supervision in groups or as an individual parental unit, counseling and supervising the child's environment (teachers, educators, counselors), family therapy, peer interventions (via the child's class), or child therapy, individually or in a group. The selection of the optimal setting should also consider problem variables as well as developmental components.

Phase 4 of the decision making facilitates the selection of suitable techniques from among the variety of verbal, nonverbal, direct, and indirect interventions available for children. Once again, this decision is influenced both by the kind of disorder and by developmental considerations. It is easier to treat emotional disorders using nonverbal techniques and behavioral disorders using verbal techniques; nonverbal techniques are better suited for younger children; and so on.

The self-control intervention that I applied, for treating and evaluating the child and for maintaining treatment outcomes, integrates cognitive and constructivist techniques via the four SCIM modules (see Figure 13.1 and Chapter 4). In applying the model, the child's problems and skill deficits and the goals of therapy should be considered.

The fifth and last phase is directed toward evaluating and maintaining treatment outcomes through the application of methods such as generalization, transfer, overlearning, practicing, charting, and relapse prevention. As described in Chapter 4, this is likewise a matter of the child's age and the type and severity of the disorder. It should be emphasized that, throughout the whole intervention process, ongoing assessment is the rule of thumb for the therapist undertaking this treatment approach.

In order to demonstrate my proposed integration of theoretical, clinical, developmental, and practical concepts and techniques, I presented seven case studies. As can be seen in Figure 13.2, the cases cover a range of ages from early childhood to adolescence. The cases of Ben and Ari relate to early childhood. Lee and Dan are at the stage of middle childhood, and Sharon, Guy, and Jacob illustrate cases of treating adolescents.

The cases also represent different childhood problems. The treatment goal of decreasing behavior is described via Dan's pain, Sharon's enuresis, and Guy's aggressiveness. The goal of increasing behavior is presented by way of Ben's mutism, Lee's traumatic response, the second part of Guys' treatment in increasing prosocial behavior and Jacob's depression and low self-esteem. The goal of removing anxiety is illustrated through Ari's anxiety, Lee's stress and anxiety, and Jacob's anxiety and depression. As can be seen, some disorders require intervention targeting more than one goal.

In presenting these cases, I tried to emphasize the children's own stories, struggles, and affective experiences, and to highlight creative techniques for helping them cope with their problems.

During this entire process of intervention, three parties are involved: the client, the therapist, and the therapy itself. Therefore, the therapeutic relationship

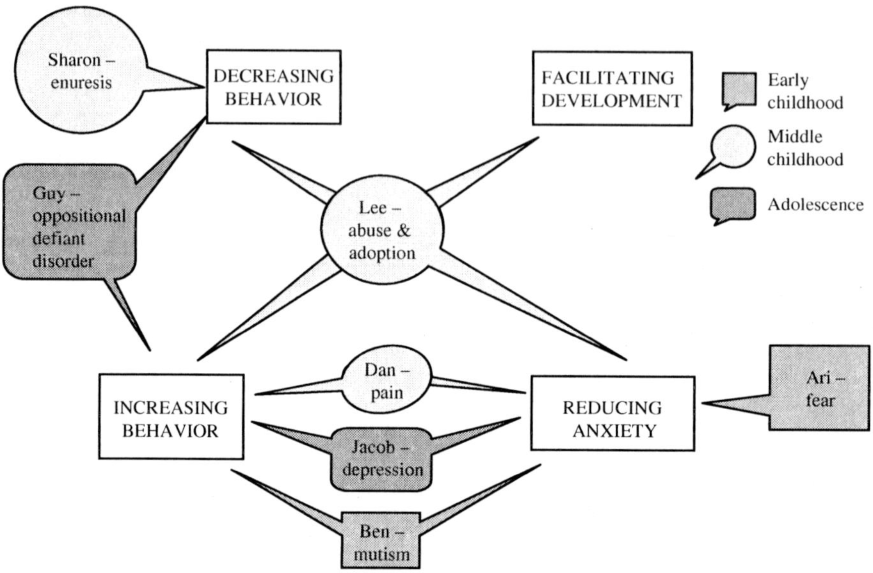

Figure 13.2 The seven case illustrations distributed by problem type and developmental stage.

itself is an important issue, comprising one of the most significant emotional experiences that children may experience. In the first part of the book, I undertook to address all three. While relating to the client, I focused on variables associated with childhood and adolescence. In discussing components such as developmental and cognitive stages, gender and emotional features, hobbies, and personal characteristics, I hoped to enhance the reader's awareness of the need to learn about the unique characteristics of the treated child. While relating to the therapist, I reviewed components such as the ability to make decisions not only in light of the therapist's skills, knowledge, and training, but also the therapist's own characteristics and leanings toward creativity. In relating to the therapy, I focused on process variables. I proposed a set of questions and considerations that can help design the intervention process in a most effective way. The next chapter elaborates on two of these components in the treatment process: one relating to the role of the therapist in flexibly applying a creative intervention, and the other focusing on the important role of the therapeutic relationship.

14

Epilogue: The Therapeutic Relationship and the Therapists's Own Creativity and Flexibility

Within the interwoven fabric laced together by the therapist, client, and intervention process, two pivotal fibers cannot be overemphasized for their impact on the therapy's final texture. These fibers, discussed here in this epilogue, constitute the therapeutic relationship and the therapist's own creativity.

THE ROLE OF THE THERAPEUTIC RELATIONSHIP IN DECISION MAKING AND INTERVENTION

In the past, the literature on cognitive and on behavioral therapy placed little emphasis on either the role of emotions in treatment or on the therapeutic relationship, focusing, rather, on types of problems and on techniques for changing behavior. Constructivist therapy, on the other hand, posited the view that therapeutic relationships comprise a markedly crucial component within the human ability to change (Mahoney, 1991). As a result, cognitive–constructivist behavioral therapists of today are far more apt to acknowledge the priority of feeling in shaping their knowing and doing (Mahoney, 1991). Clinicians nowadays are seeking out ways to better understand affective processes in order to learn how to deal with, handle, and change emotions. The growing recognition of the importance of emotion has led to an increased accentuation of internal processes and a sharper focus on affects, and, consequently, a burgeoning emphasis on treatment processes and therapeutic relationships (Mahoney, 1991, 1995).

The therapeutic relationship can be seen as a framework that encompasses the entire treatment process. This relationship is conceived as the organizing feature via which collaboration between therapist and client is built. Collaboration embodies the major component of the intervention process, which is crucial for the application of assessment, intervention, evaluation, and maintenance. A good therapeutic relationship creates trust, openness, and a willingness to cooperate. This relationship is a prerequisite even in the earliest stages of assessment in order to achieve an efficient assessment process, the reliable collection of data from all parties involved, an accurate diagnosis, and appropriate decision making regarding whether the client needs therapy. Without a good therapeutic relationship, the therapist will find it very difficult to foster the client's open expression, acknowledgment, and sharing of his or her problems and concerns, or even to secure the client's agreement that the therapist contact and obtain information from the environment.

The influence of the therapist–client relationship is even more central when it comes to the process of intervention. Therapy is not only a lengthy process and therefore subject to changes in the character and intensity of the relationship, but also requires the child as well as the therapist to confront and cope with difficulties, weaknesses, and deficits. Good therapeutic relationships help the child persevere during what may be difficult, painful, or frightening therapeutic processes. It encourages the client's investment of effort into the process of change. It also helps empower the client to become independent. Therapeutic relationships should include supportive elements, components that serve an educating and training function, and emotional ingredients that enable the client to cope with perceived threats and obstacles.

Different researchers have addressed the importance of therapeutic relationships in cognitive and constructivist interventions. The behavioral component of the therapeutic relationship is reflected in Bandura's (1969) view of its important role in creating influential social processes. The basic feature for conceiving the therapist thus is one of a model to be observed and learned from, and to help design positive expectations. A more cognitive view asserts the necessity of relationships to afford empiricist collaboration and facilitate the change process (Beck, 1976), or conceptualizes therapeutic relationships as a laboratory for new experiences (Safran & Segal, 1990). Constructivists view the therapeutic relationship in the context of personal experiences and growth. This relationship is shared between client and therapist as a mutual emotional experience (Mahoney, 1991, 1995). Rosenbaum and Ronen (1998) presented their view of cognitive–constructivist therapy. They emphasized that the therapeutic relationship is influenced by expectations, ways of thinking, and schemata that both the therapist and client bring to the therapeutic interaction.

With children, the therapeutic relationship plays more diverse functions than in adult therapy. The unique nature of the therapeutic relationship in child therapy lies primarily in the fact that children will not remain in therapy if they do not like the therapist. A parallel may be drawn from children's functioning in their studies: Young students invest much more effort and obtain far better results if they like their teachers. In addition, as mentioned earlier, children's different perceptions of time and cognitive limitations require that therapy provide more short-term, concrete achievements and rewards. For these reasons, child therapists must embrace more roles than do adult therapists, including teaching, modeling, guiding, and direct helping. In addition to the classic supportive role and to the function of mediator between stress and behavior, child therapists may also provide direct, concrete assistance as when working to improve homework competence and may also act in a preventive capacity, as a model for new roles, and as a laboratory for experiencing and experimentation.

One of the problematic aspects of therapeutic relationships in child therapy revolves around the fact that the child therapist treats more than one client. The child is not the only client in his or her environment being treated. Child therapists must by definition also be involved with members of the child's environment such as the parents, teachers, family, and peers. Therapeutic relationships in those settings as well should be of fundamental concern to the therapist, in order to create good collaboration with the entire client system.

A good therapeutic relationship enables the therapist to initially make an appropriate decision about the need for therapy, and to determine the best means for applying therapy so as to enlist the child's motivation and compliance with treatment goals. Yet, such a relationship is crucial not only in initiating the process of intervention but also throughout that process as a major tool to help the child change, accept, or overcome the problems at hand. As can be seen in Figure 14.1, the ability to adequately and efficiently assess and treat children and adolescents is, first and foremost, a matter of being able to create an effectual alliance with the child. The therapist must initially consider the individual child's characteristics: hobbies, unique nature, motivation, support systems, and so on. All of these components directly influence the way the child will collaborate with the process of assessment and intervention and put effort into creating change. Together with the child variables, therapist variables come into play. Components such as personality, training, gender, creativity, and flexibility will affect the therapist's style in creating a good alliance and a trusting, working relationship. Likewise, such components impinge on the degree to which the therapist will collaborate with the child, allowing the child to actively participate and contribute during the process of assessment and intervention.

An awareness of these two sets of variables, the client and the therapist variables, can both be useful for assessing, for treating, and for evaluating and maintaining treatment outcomes. The assessment and intervention process can be best directed only if a good collaborative atmosphere and a good relationship develop between the two. This collaboration enables them, together, to obtain information, analyze knowledge, define goals and means for treatment, and interpret achievements.

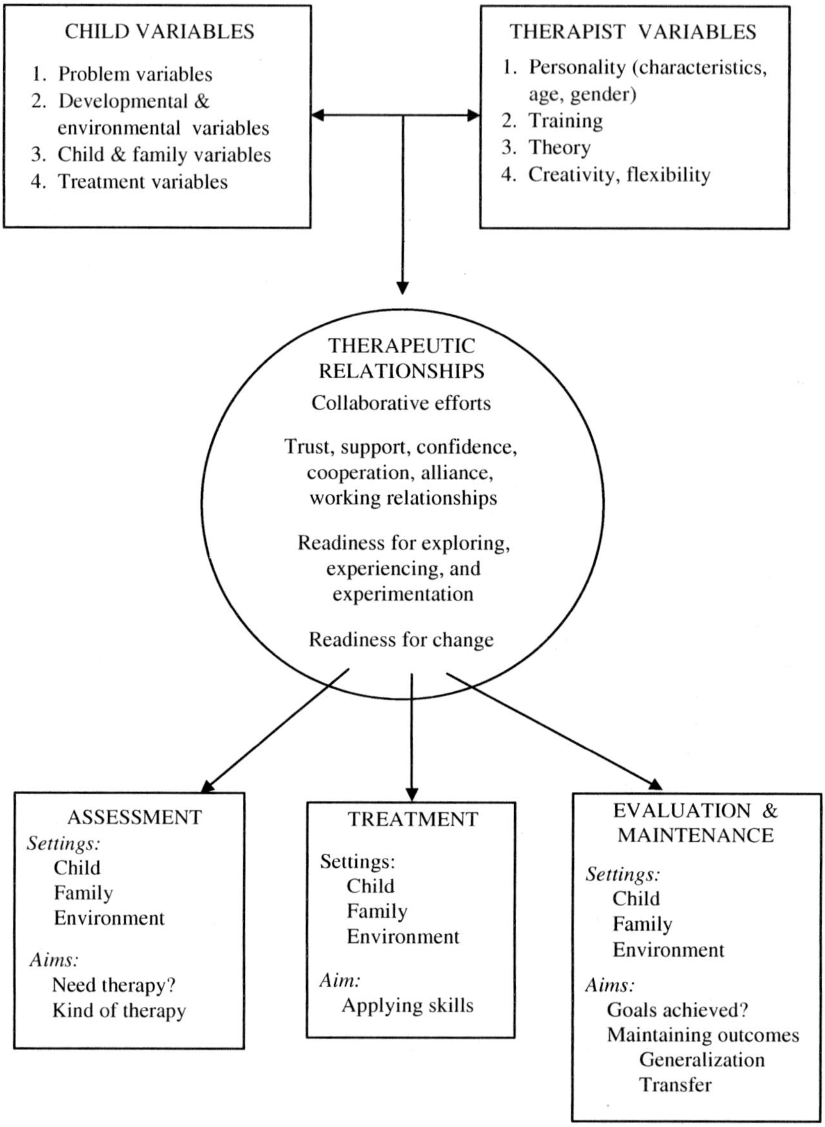

Figure 14.1 Variables affecting the process of intervention.

In sum, the application of cognitive–constructivist therapy with children consists of a process of decision making regarding what is needed for the specific child, with the specific problem, in the specific situation. Only via the establishment of a good therapeutic relationship can the entire assessment and treatment process be conducted, to obtain the maximal benefit from all of the phases described in Chapter 4. Another crucial component to ensure maximal results from therapeutic intervention involves the attempt to arrive at the best match possible between the client's needs and the therapist's strategies and practices. This match necessitates, obviously, that the therapist be finely attuned to the client, exercise the required knowledge and expertise, and furnish the optimal conditions for a good therapeutic alliance. Yet, the therapist's willingness to take risks, be daring and open to new experiences, and go with the flow initiated by the client into hitherto uncharted territories (for this therapist) appears to provide the strongest likelihood that an optimal match with the client will be obtained, leading to the most rapid and effective changes in the client.

THERAPIST FLEXIBILITY AND CREATIVITY

In designing their intervention processes, therapists should view their theoretical approach as the white dividing lines drawn on the road, which help drivers discern the center and edges of the road, and take care not to cross them. The driver is free to choose the destination, the kind of car to buy (which brand, automatic versus manual gear), and how to increase safety through precautionary measures (seat belts, regular check-ups of breaks, lights, etc). To some extent, as long as he or she does not disregard the permissible limits (of speed and traffic signs), the driver has freedom of choice, in determining, for example, how fast to drive, or how far from the white line to maintain the car. The driver can decide which roads, detours, or shortcuts to take along the way, whether to use familiar traffic routes or to experiment with new and creative ones. So, there are a handful of decisions the driver can make, despite being limited by laws and regulations.

Like the driver, the therapist has the freedom to choose the session-to-session content of therapy, the way the process progresses, and the means and modes to help children change. Within the accepted limits, the therapist has a range of decisions to make and a great deal of flexibility. This book has aimed to foster therapists' ability to systematically consider the multitude of options and issues involved in child referrals, as well as to integrate creative modes into their regular intervention practices.

We should not adapt our clients to our own beliefs or models. Rather, we should change, adapt, and fit our interventions to the clients' needs. Careful attention to the child's way of communicating will point us toward the most effective means of intervention. If the child uses metaphors or imagination, this can open a window to communication with the child, suggesting the efficacy of these modes in therapy. If the child enjoys drawing or playing, it will be easier to meet the child on that ground.

Child treatment is a combination of art and skills. Combining both of these together will enable us to travel the maze of routes we need to reach our destination and end our journey successfully.

The effective therapist is not necessarily one who knows a great number of creative means and methods or one who is highly experienced in one particular approach such as the cognitive–constructivist orientation. Rather, the effective therapist is one who demonstrates the ability to use his or her own feelings as a tool, to connect with the child, to attend to the child's pace and style, and to be sensitive and accepting of the emotions he or she encounters in the child. Only a therapist who is understanding and accepting of the child's subjective world and emotions, and who dares to listen and acknowledge his or her own feelings, can develop the flexibility and the proficiency to introduce creative modes appropriately.

As therapists, we are accustomed to listening to an endless variety of people, problems, and configurations. We are keenly attuned to even the slightest deviance or idiosyncrasy when conducting our intake assessments, in order to understand the complex individuality of each client. However, in designing interventions, many therapists' openness stops there. Commonly, therapists tend to bring their most familiar, customary, even habitual intervention method to the treatment room and tend to apply it in almost every case.

We should not fear customizing and personalizing our methods to our individual clients, especially to the wondrous intricacy of childhood and adolescence. Yet, many therapists do.

I believe this reluctance stems mainly from unfamiliarity and from trepidation about unconventionality or nonconformity. Yes, some of us were trained or had practice in one major therapeutic approach, and the confines of this background experience can be difficult to breach. Only the occasional training or supervision program has more than a passing reference to a cognitive–constructivist viewpoint and the creative integration of various techniques. Furthermore, seldom indeed do therapists and students of psychotherapy experiment and experience firsthand the range of techniques available for children.

Several years ago, in the master's program for social work at Tel Aviv University, I began to regularly include such experiential practice in the curriculum for students who were already doing practical work with children in different treatment settings. I believe that the integration of experiential methods into the theoretical curriculum is an urgent, substantive need for students of therapeutic intervention. My underlying assumption is that these social work students can become more effective, attuned therapists if they allow themselves to recapture what it was for them to be a young girl or boy and if they experience a wide range of therapeutic techniques on the receiving end, rather than the dispensing end.

I often begin by asking students to make drawings using different media and to portray themselves, their families, and the group of students in the class. I bring in, among others, an art therapist to work with them on sculpturing and thus to acquaint them with this expressive technique of using the body for communication, individually and with small and large groups.

One of my early attempts to introduce such experiences into the coursework proved very difficult. Although I worked hard to avoid transforming the class into dynamic group therapy or highlighting their personal problems, the students were embarrassed, flustered, uncooperative, and resistant. They had expected theoretical discourse and felt vulnerable and insecure. They did not want to expose themselves to one another or to me, worrying about criticism.

I explained that therapy cannot be learned from afar, just as swimming cannot be learned from a correspondence course. A person who cannot work on himself or herself through practicing activities such as drawing, dancing, and so on, cannot feel secure in the treatment room performing such exercises with children.

I designated these experiences as experimentation within a laboratory, to enable learning new skills. I emphasized that the students might see personal issues arise, but that they could deal with these on their own time at home. I redefined their insecurity, not as simply a personal vulnerability or interpersonal fear, but as a lack of confidence due to inexperience and unfamiliarity with these new skills and with the use of themselves as the therapeutic tool of choice.

After a period of hesitation and disconcertion, the students "jumped right into the water." They began to really enjoy the experiential exercises. They were soon able to relate stories and anecdotes about how they were applying these exercises and techniques to their work in the field. These efforts significantly contributed to their understanding of the youngsters they were treating.

At times, the group did enter the ground of private concerns. In one activity, the students were asked to model themselves in children's play dough, while keeping their eyes closed. One heavy-set student said she wanted to share something personal evoked by this exercise. She said she was very self-conscious about her body and that, even with her eyes closed, it was obvious from her self-portrait that she felt her large body was disproportionate to her small head. The group supported her, complimenting her on her disclosure and on her congeniality as a colleague. They also disagreed with her perception of disproportionality and assured her that her weight or size were not factors in their rapport. She cried, and told the class that this had been a significant positive experience for her.

Yet, most of the time our work focused on therapy-related insights. For example, the group was asked to walk around the classroom and greet one another without words. Most of the students reported afterwards that this was an extremely difficult exercise. They realized how much they rely on words and how hard it is to touch one another physically. A significant discussion emerged about how different children are in relation to physical contact, how much simpler and more natural touch is for them, how much adults have become inhibited in this domain, and how touch should or should not be integrated in the treatment room.

My own experience teaching this course reinforced for me the profound value of learning a creative openness and a wide variety of verbal, nonverbal, direct, and indirect techniques "on one's own skin." I subsequently included in my entire course curricula the opportunity for each student of psychotherapy to experience drawing, metaphors, imagination, movement, and so on with himself or herself before beginning the process of analyzing these drawings and other tools as applied with clients. I might add that these course components have proven very popular among the students over the years, further reinforcing my conviction of its importance for professional development.

I came to the conclusion that learning to be a child therapist is difficult, if not impossible, without working on the significance of being a child, and on the unique differences between adults and children. Flushing out the small details is well facilitated by these hands-on experiences, such as sitting down low to be at the child's height, speaking simply and clearly, getting to know the child's language, and even selecting appropriate clothing.

With children, we cannot hide behind our desks, our sophisticated words, our big theories, and our power suits. We need to roll up our sleeves, get down on the floor, and dare to do it ourselves. We need to meet that specific child or teenager where he or she is, and to devise the best ways to help, using our cognitive–constructivist orientation, our repertoire of creative techniques, our open and flexible attitude, and most importantly, ourselves as the most significant tool in therapy, the tool that guides us to select and apply diverse theories and techniques at different intervals in therapy.

References

Achenbach, T. M. (1985). *Assessment and taxonomy of child and adolescent psychopathology*. Beverly Hills, CA: Sage.

Achenbach, T. M. (1993). Implications of multiaxial empirically based assessment for behavior therapy with children. *Behavior Therapy, 24*, 91–116.

Achenbach, T. M. & Edelbrock, C. S. (1983). *Manual for the child behavior checklist and revised child behavior profile*. Burlington: University of Vermont.

Albano, A. M., Chorpita, B. F., & Barlow, D. H. (1996). Childhood anxiety disorders. In E. J. Mash & R. A. Barkley (Eds.), *Child psychopathology* (pp. 196–241). New York: Guilford Press.

Alcazar, A. I. R., Rodriguez, J. O., & Sanchez, M. J. (1999). Meta-analysis de-las intervenciones conductuales de la enuresis en Espana. (Meta analysis of interventions conducted on enuresis in Spain). *Anales-de-Psicologia, 15*, 157–167.

Alexander, D. W. (1999). *Children changed by trauma. A healing guide*. Oakland, CA: New Harbinger.

Alexander, J. F., Holtzworth-Munroe, A., & Jameson, P. B. (1994). The process and outcome of marital and family therapy research: Review and evaluation. In A. E. Bergin & L. Garfield (Eds.), *Handbook of psychotherapy and behavior change* (4th ed., pp. 595–630). New York: Wiley.

Alford, B. A. & Beck, A. T. (1997). *The integrative power of cognitive therapy*. New York: Guilford Press.

Ambrosini, P. J. (2000). A review of pharmacotherapy of major depression in children and adolescents. *Psychiatric Services, 5*, 627–633.

American Psychiatric Association. (1994). *Diagnostic and statistical manual of mental disorders: DSM-IV* (4th ed.) Washington, DC: Author.

Anderson, J. C. (1994). Epidemiological issues. In T. Ollendick, N. King & W. Yule (Eds.), *International handbook of phobic and anxiety disorders in children and adolescents* (pp. 43–66). New York: Plenum.

Anderson, J. C., Williams, S., McGee, R., & Silva, P. A. (1987). DSM-III disorders in preadolescent children: Prevalence in a large sample from general population. *Archive of Genetic Psychiatry, 44*, 69–76.

Angold, A., Weissman, M., Merikangas, J. K., Prusoff, B., Wickramaratne, P., Gammon, G., & Warner, B. (1987). Parent and child reports of depressive symptoms in children at low and high risk of depression. *Journal of Child Psychology and Psychiatry, 28*, 901–915.

Axline, V. (1947). *Play therapy*. Boston: Houghton Mifflin.

Ayllon, T., Smith, D., & Rogers, M. (1970). Behavioral management of school phobia. *Journal of Behavior Therapy and Experimental Psychiatry, 1*, 125–138.

Azrin, N. H. & Foxx, R. M. (1974). *Toilet training in less than a day*. New York: Simon & Schuster.

Azrin, N. H., Sneed, T. J., & Foxx, R. M. (1974). Dry-bed training: Rapid elimination of childhood enuresis. *Behaviour Research and Therapy, 12*, 147–156.

Azrin, N. H. & Thiens, P. M. (1978). Rapid elimination of childhood enuresis. *Behavior Therapy, 9*, 342–354.

Bailey, V. (1998). Conduct disorders in young children. In P. Graham (Ed.), *Cognitive behaviour therapy with children and families* (pp. 95–109). Cambridge: University Press.

Bakwin, H. (1971). Enuresis in twins. *American Journal of Diseases of Children, 121*, 222–225.

Bandura, A. (1969). *Principles of behavior modification.* New York: Holt, Rinehart & Winston.

Bandura, A. (1997). *Self-efficacy: The exercise of control.* New York: W. H. Freeman.

Bandura, A., Caprara, G. V., Barbaranelli, C., & Pastorelli, C. (2001). Sociocognitive self-regulatory mechanisms governing transgressive behavior. *Journal of Personality and Social Behavior, 80*, 125–135.

Barrett, P. M. (2000). Treatment of childhood anxiety: Developmental aspects. *Clinical Psychology Review, 20*, 479–494.

Barrios, B. A. & Hartman, D. P. (1988). Fears and anxieties. In E. J. Mash & L. G. Terdal (Eds.), *Behavioral assessment of childhood disorders* (pp. 196–262). New York: Guilford Press.

Barron, F. (1988). Putting creativity to work. In R. Sternberg (Ed.), *The nature of creativity* (pp. 76–98). Cambridge, UK: Cambridge University Press.

Beck, A. T. (1963). Thinking and depression. *Archives of General Psychiatry, 9*, 324–333.

Beck, A. T. (1976). *Cognitive therapy and the emotional disorders.* New York: Meridian.

Beck, A. T., Emery, G., & Greenberg, R. L. (1985). *Anxiety disorders and phobias.* New York: Basic Books.

Beck, A. T., Freeman, A., & Associates (1990). *Cognitive therapy of personality disorders.* New York: Guilford Press.

Beck, A. T., Rush, A. J., Shaw, B. F., & Emery, G. (1979). *Cognitive therapy of depression.* New York: Guilford Press.

Bellver-Cebria, V. (1999). Tratamiento de la disfemia y yenuresis en el marco escolar. (Treatment of stuttering and enuresis in the school framework). *Analisis-y Modification-de-Conducta, 25*, 955–969.

Bemporad, J. (1978). Psychotherapy of depression in children and adolescents. In S. Arieti & J. Bemporad (Eds.), *Severe and mild depression: A psychotherapeutic approach* (pp. 344–357). New York: Basic Books.

Beres, D. (1966). Superego and depression. In R. M. Lowenstein, M. Scherr, & A. J. Solnit (Eds.), *Psychoanalytics: A general psychology* (pp. 479–498). New York: International University Press.

Berg, I., Forsythe, I., & McGuire, R. (1982). Response of bed wetting to the enuresis alarm: Influence of psychiatric disturbance and maximum functional bladder capacity. *Archive of Disease in Childhood, 57*, 394–396.

Biederman, J., Faraone, S. V., Hirshfeld-Becker, D. R., Friedman, D., Robin, J. A., & Rosenbaum, J. F. (2001). Patterns of psychopathology and dysfunction in high-risk children of parents with panic disorder and major depression. *American Journal of Psychiatry, 158*, 49–57.

Bierman, K. L. & Furman, W. (1984). The effects of social skills training and peer involvement on the social adjustment of preadolescents. *Child Development, 55*, 151–162

Black, B. & Ude, T. W. (1992). Elective mutism as a variant of social phobia. *Journal of Academic Child and Adolescent Psychiatry, 31*, 1090–1094.

Blackwell, B. & Currah, J. (1973). The psychopharmacology of nocturnal enuresis. In I. Kolvin, R. C. MacKeith, & S. R. Meadow (Eds.), *Bladder control and enuresis* (pp. 231–257). London: Heinemann.

Bowen, K. (2000). Child abuse and domestic violence in families of children seen for suspected sexual abuse. *Clinical Pediatrics, 39*, 33–40.

Bowlby, J. (1969). *Attachment and loss* (Vol. 1). New York: Basic Books.

Bowlby, J. (1973). *Attachment and loss* (Vol. 2). New York: Basic Books.

Bowlby, J. (1988). Developmental psychiatry comes of age. In *A secure base.* New York: Basic Books.

Brady, E. U. & Kendall, P. C. (1992). Comorbidity of anxiety and depression in children and adolescents. *Psychological Bulletin, 111*, 244–255.

Brandell, J. R. (1992). Psychotherapy of a traumatized 10-year-old boy: Theoretical issues and clinical considerations. *Smith College Studies in Social Work, 62*, 123–138.

Brigham, T. A., Hopper, A. J., Shaw, B. F., & Emery, G. (1979). *Cognitive therapy of depression.* New York: Guilford Press.

Campbell, S. (1990). *Behavior problems in preschool children.* New York: Guilford Press.

Carlsen, M. B. (1995). Meaning-making and creative aging. In R. A. Neimeyer & M. J. Mahoney (Eds.), *Constructivism in psychotherapy* (pp. 127–153). Washington, DC: American Psychological Association.

Carlson, J. S., Kratochwill, T. R., & Johnson, H. F. (1999). Sertraline treatment of 5 children diagnosed with selective mutism: A single-case research trial. *Journal of Child and Adolescence Psychopharmacology, 9,* 293–306.

Clark, D. A. (1995). Perceived limitations of standard cognitive therapy: A consideration of efforts to revise Beck's theory and therapy. *Journal of Cognitive Psychotherapy: An International Quarterly, 9,* 153–172.

Cohen, J. S., Mannarino, A. P., Berliner, L., & Deblinger, E. (2000). Trauma focused cognitive behavioral therapy for children and adolescence: An empirical update. *Journal of Interpersonal Violence, 15,* 1202–1223.

Conners, C. K. (1969). A teacher rating scale for use in drug studies with children. *American Journal of Psychiatry, 126,* 884–888.

Copeland, A. P. (1982). Individual difference factors in children's self-management: Toward individualized treatment. In P. Karoly & F. H. Kanfer (Eds.), *Self-management and behavior change. From theory to practice* (pp. 207–239). New York: Pergamon Press.

Cowen, E. L. (1980). The wooing of primary prevention strategy. *American Journal of Community Psychology, 8,* 258–284.

Crick, N. R. & Dodge, K. A. (1994). A review and reformulation of social information-processing mechanisms in children's social adjustment. *Psychological Bulletin, 115,* 74–101.

Crumley, F. H. (1990). The masquerade of mutism. *Journal of Academic Child and Adolescent Psychiatry, 29,* 318–319.

Csikszentmihalyi, M. (1966). *Creativity: Flow and the psychology of discovery and invention.* New York: Harper Collins.

Cytryn, L. & McKnew, D. H. (1974). Factors influencing the changing clinical expression of the depressive process in children. *American Journal of Psychiatry, 131,* 879–881.

De Jong, G. A. (1973). Epidemiology of enuresis: A survey of the literature. In L. Kolvin, R. C. MacKeith, & S. R. Meadow (Eds.), *Bladder control and enuresis* (pp. 66–69). London: Heinemann.

Doleys, D. M. (1977). Behavioral treatments for nocturnal enuresis in children: A review of the recent literature. *Psychological Bulletin, 84,* 30–54.

Doleys, D. M., Ciminero, A. R., Tollison, J. W., Williams, C. L., & Wells, K. C. (1977). Dry bed training and retention control training: A comparison. *Behavior Therapy, 8,* 541–548.

Donovan, C. L. & Spence, S. H. (2000). Prevention of childhood anxiety disorders. *Clinical Psychology Review, 24,* 509–531.

Dow, S. P., Stones, B. C., Scheib, B., Moss, S. H. M., & Leonard, H. L. (1995). Practical guidelines for the assessment and treatment of selective mutism. *Journal of American Academy of Child & Adolescent Psychiatry, 34,* 836–846.

Dubrow, N. & Garbarino, J. (1988). Living in the war zone: Mothers and young children in a public housing project. *Child Welfare, 68,* 3–20.

Durlak, J. A., Fuhrman, T., & Lampman, C. (1991). Effectiveness of cognitive-behavior therapy for maladaptive children: A meta-analysis. *Psychological Bulletin, 110,* 204–214.

Dush, D. M., Hirt, M. L., & Schroeder, H. E. (1989). Self-statement modification in the treatment of child behavior disorders: A meta-analysis. *Psychological Bulletin, 106,* 97–106.

Elbedour, S., Shulman, S., & Kedem, P. (1997). Children's fears: Cultural and developmental perspectives. *Behavior Research & Therapy, 35,* 491–496.

Elias, M. J., Gara, M., Ubriaco, M., Rothbaum, P., Clabby, J. F., & Schuyler, T. (1986). Impact of a preventive social problem solving intervention on children's coping with middle stressors. *American Journal of Community Psychology, 14*, 259–275.

Ellis, A. (1962). *Reason and emotion in psychotherapy*. New York: Lyle Stuart.

Essau, C. A., Conradt, J., & Petermann, F. (1999). Prevalence, comorbidity and psychosocial impairment of somatoform disorders in adolescence. *Psychology, Health and Medicine, 4*, 169–180.

Eyberg, S. M. (1980). Eyberg behavior inventory. *Journal of Clinical Child Psychology, 9*, 29.

Faravelli, C., Salvatori, S., Galassi, F., & Aiazzi, L. (1997). Epidemiology of somatoform disorders: A community survey in Florence. *Social and Psychiatric Epidemiology, 32*, 24–29.

Feldman, D. H. (1988). Creativity: Dreams, insights, and transformations. In R. Sternberg (Ed.), *The nature of creativity* (pp. 271–297). Cambridge, UK: Cambridge University Press.

Fielding, D. M. (1980). The response of day and night wetting children and children who wet only at night to retention control training and the enuresis alarm. *Behaviour Research and Therapy, 18*, 305–317.

Fielding, D. M. & Doleys, D. M. (1988). Elimination problems: Enuresis and encopresis. In E. J. Mash & L. G. Terdal (Eds.), *Behavioral assessment of childhood disorders* (pp. 586–623). New York: Guilford Press.

Finley, W. W., Besserman, R. L., Benntt, I. F., Clapp, R. K., & Finley, P. M. (1973). The effect of continuous intermittent and "placebo" reinforcement on the effectiveness of the conditioning treatment for enuresis nocturna. *Behavior Research and Therapy, 11*, 289–297.

Ford, J. D., Racusin, R., Ellis, C. G., Daviss, W. B., Reiser, J., Fleischer, A., & Thomas, J. (2000). Child maltreatment, other trauma exposure and posttraumatic symptomatology among children with oppositional defiant and attention deficit hyperactive disorders. *Child Maltreatment Journal of the American Professional Society on the Abuse of Children, 5*, 205–217.

Fordyce, W. E. (1976). *Behavioral methods for chronic pain and illness*. St Louis: Mosby.

Forehand, R. & McMahon, R. J. (1981). *Helping the non-compliant child: A clinician's guide to effective parent training*. New York: Guilford Press.

Forehand, R. & Weirson, M. (1993). The role of developmental factors in planning behavioral intervention for children: Disruptive behavior as an example. *Behavior Therapy, 24*, 117–141.

Freud, A. & Burlingham, D. (1943). *War and children*. New York: Ernest Willard.

Freud, S. (1957). Mourning and melancholia. In J. Strachey (Ed. and Trans.), *Standard edition of the complete psychological works of Sigmund Freud* (Vol. 14, pp. 243–258). London: Hogarth Press.

Fritz, G. K., Fritsch, S., & Hagino, O. (1997). Somatoform disorders in children and adolescents: A review of the past 10 years. *Journal of the American Academy of Child and Adolescent Psychiatry, 36*, 1329–1338.

Furman, E. (1986). On trauma: When is the death of a parent traumatic? *Psychoanalytic Study of the Child, 41*, 191–208.

Gambrill, E. (1990). *Critical thinking in clinical practice*. San Francisco: Jossey-Bass.

Gambrill, E. (1995a). Behavioral social work: Past, present and future. *Research on Social Work Practice, 5*, 460–484.

Gambrill, E. (1995b). Helping shy, socially anxious, and lonely adults: A skill based contextual approach. In W. O'Donohue & L. Krasner (Eds.), *Handbook of psychological skill training: Clinical techniques and applications*. Boston: Allyn & Bacon.

Gambrill, E. Thomas, E. J., & Carter, R. D. (1971). Procedure for sociobehavioral practice in open settings. *Social Work, 16*, 51–62.

Garbarino, J., Kostelny, K., & Dubrow, N. (1991). What children can tell us about living in danger. *American Psychologist, 46*, 376–383.

Garmezy, N. & Rutter, M. (1985). Acute reactions to stress. In M. Rutter & L. Hersov (Eds.), *Child and adolescent psychiatry: Modern approaches* (2nd ed., pp. 152–176). Oxford: Blackwell.

Goldman, J., L'Engle Stein, C., & Guerry, S. (1983). *Psychological methods of child assessment*. New York: Brunner/Mazel.

Gordon, S. L. (1989). The socialization of children's emotions: Emotional culture, competence, and exposure. In C. Saarni & P. L. Harris (Eds.), *Children's understanding of emotion* (pp. 319–344). New York: Cambridge University Press.

Graham, P. (1994). Prevention. In M. Rutter, E. Taylor, & L. Hersov (Eds.), *Child and adolescent psychiatry: Modern approaches* (3rd ed., pp. 815–828). Oxford: Blackwell.

Graziano, A. M. (1978). Behavior therapy. In B. B. Wolman & A. O. Ross (Eds.). *Handbook of treatment of mental disorders in childhood and adolescence.* Englewood Cliffs, NJ: Prentice Hall.

Graziano, A. M., Monney, K. C., Hurber, C., & Ignasiak, D. (1979). Self-control instruction for children's fear-reduction. *Journal of Behavior Therapy and Experimental Psychology, 10*, 221–227.

Greenberg, L. S. & Safran, J. D. (1987). *Emotion in psychotherapy.* New York: Guilford Press.

Gresham, F. M. (1981). Social skills training with handicapped children: A review. *Review of Educational Research, 51*, 139–176.

Gross, A. M. & Drabman, R. S. (1982). Teaching self-recording, self-evaluation, and self-reward to non-clinic children and adolescents. In P. K. Karoly & F. H. Kanfer (Eds.), *Self-management and behavior change: From theory to practice* (pp. 285–314). New York: Pergamon Press.

Guidano, V. F. (1995). A constructivist outline of human knowing processes. In M. J. Mahoney (Ed.), *Cognitive and constructive psychotherapies: Theory, research, and practice* (pp. 89–102). New York: Springer.

Haggerty, J. J. (1983). The psychosomatic family: An overview. *Psychosomatics, 24*, 615–623.

Hannan, A. P., Rapee, R. M., & Hudson, J. L. (2000). The prevention of depression in children: A pilot study. *Behaviour Change, 17*, 78–83.

Herbert, M. (1987). *Conduct disorders of childhood and adolescence: A social learning perspective* (2nd ed.). Chichester, UK: Wiley.

Hersen, M. & Bellack, A. S. (1981). *Behavioral assessment.* New York: Pergamon Press.

Hodges, K., Gordon, Y., & Lennon, M. P. (1990). Parent–child agreement on symptoms assessed via clinical research interview for children: The child assessment schedule (CAS). *Journal of Child Psychiatry, 31*, 427–436.

Hollon, S. D. & Beck, A. T. (1994). Cognitive and cognitive behavioral therapies. In A. E. Bergin & S. L. Garfield (Eds.), *Handbook of psychotherapy and behavior change* (4th ed., pp. 428–466). New York: Wiley

Houts, A. C. (1991). Nocturnal enuresis as a biobehavioral problem. *Behavior Therapy, 22*, 133–151.

Houts, A. C., Berman, J. S., & Abramson, H. (1994). Effectiveness of psychological and pharmacological treatments for nocturnal enuresis. *Journal of Consulting and Clinical Psychology, 62*, 737–745.

Howard, B. L. & Kendall, P. C. (1996). Cognitive–behavioral family therapy for anxiety-disordered children: A multiple-baseline evaluation. *Cognitive Therapy & Research, 20*, 423–443.

Hughes, J. N. (1993). Behavior therapy. In T. R. Kratochwill & R. J. Morris (Eds.), *Handbook of psychotherapy with children and adolescents* (pp. 185–220). Boston: Allyn & Bacon.

Hurwich, C. (1992). *Late-life potential.* Panel discussion presented at the annual meeting of the American Society on Aging, San Diego, CA.

Jacobson, T. (1995). Case study: Is selective mutism a manifestation of dissociative identity disorder? *Journal of American Academy of Child and Adolescent Psychiatry, 34*, 863–866.

Jersild, A. T. (1968). *Child psychology* (6th ed.). Englewood Cliffs, NJ: Prentice Hall.

Jersild, A. T. & Holmes, F. (1935). *Children's fear.* New York: Columbia University Press.

Johnson, S. B. (1980). Enuresis. In R. Daitzman (Ed.), *Clinical behavior therapy and behavior modification* (pp. 81–142). New York: Garland.

Jones, H. G. (1960). The behavioural treatment of enuresis nocturnal. In H. J. Eysenck (Ed.), *Behaviour therapy and the neuroses* (pp. 377–402). Oxford: Pergamon Press.

Kanfer, F. H., Karoly, P., & Newman, P. (1975). Reduction of children's fear of dark by competence-related and situational threat-related verbal cues. *Journal of Consulting and Clinical Psychology, 43*, 251–258.

Kanfer, F. H. & Philips, J. S. (1970). *Learning foundation of behavior therapy.* New York: Wiley.

Kanfer, F. H. & Schefft, B. K. (1988). *Guiding the process of therapeutic change.* Champaign, IL: Research Press.

Karoly, P. & Kanfer, F. H. (Eds.). (1982). *Self-management and behavior change: From theory to practice.* New York: Pergamon Press.

Kaslow, N. J., Rehm, L. P., Pollack, S. L., & Siegal, W. (1988). Attributional style and self-control behavior in depressed and nondepressed children and their parents. *Journal of Abnormal Child Psychology, 16*, 163–175.

Kazdin, A. E. (1982). *Single-case research design: Methods for clinical and applied setting.* New York: Oxford University Press.

Kazdin, A. E. (1987). *Conduct disorders in childhood and adolescence.* Newbury Park, CA: Sage.

Kazdin, A. E. (1988a). *Child psychotherapy: Development and identifying effective treatments.* New York: Pergamon Press.

Kazdin, A. E. (1988b). Childhood depression. In E. J. Mash & L. G. Terdal (Eds.), *Behavioral assessment of childhood disorders* (2nd ed., pp. 157–195). New York: Guilford Press.

Kazdin, A. E. (1994a). Methodology, design, and evaluation in psychotherapy research. In A. E. Bergin & S. L. Garfield (Eds.), *Handbook of psychotherapy and behavior change* (4th ed., pp. 19–71). New York: Wiley.

Kazdin, A. E. (1994b). Psychotherapy for children and adolescents. In A. E. Bergin & S. L. Garfield (Eds.), *Handbook of psychotherapy and behavior change* (4th ed., pp. 543–594). New York: Wiley.

Kazdin, A. E. (1998). Psychosocial treatments for conduct disorder in children. In D. E. Nathan & J. M. Gorman (Eds.), *A guide to treatments that work* (pp. 65–89). New York: Oxford University Press.

Kazdin, A. E., Esveldt-Dawson, K. French, N. H., & Unis, A. S. (1987). Problem solving skills training and relationship therapy in the treatment of antisocial child behavior. *Journal of Consulting and Clinical Psychology, 55*, 76–85.

Kazdin, A. E., Siegal, T. C., & Bass, D. (1990). Drawing upon clinical practice to inform research on child and adolescent psychotherapy: A survey of practitioners. *Professional Psychology: Research and Practice, 21*, 189–198.

Kelly, G. A. (1955). *The psychology of personal constructs.* New York: Norton.

Kendall, P. C. (1993). Cognitive-behavioral therapies with youth: Guiding theory, current status, and emerging developments. *Journal of Consulting and Clinical Psychology, 61*, 235–247.

Kendall, P. C. (1994). Treating anxiety disorders in youth: Results of a randomized clinical trial. *Journal of Consulting and Clinical Psychology, 62*, 100–110.

Kendall P. C & Braswell, L. (1985). *Cognitive-behavioral therapy for impulsive children.* New York: Guilford Press.

Kendall, P. C. & Chu, B. C. (2000). Retrospective self-reports of therapist flexibility in a manual-based treatment for youths with anxiety disorders. *Journal of Clinical Child Psychology, 29*, 209–220.

Kendall, P. C., Kortlander, E., Chansky, T. E., & Brady, E. U. (1992). Comorbidity of anxiety and depression in youth: Treatment implications. *Journal of Consulting and Clinical Psychology, 60*, 869–880.

Kendall, P. C. & Wilcox, L. E. (1980). Cognitive–behavioral treatment for impulsivity: Concrete versus conceptual training in non-self-controlled problem children. *Journal of Consulting and Clinical Psychology, 48*, 80–91.

Kendall-Tackett, K. A., Williams, L. M., & Finkerlhor, D. (1993). Impact of sexual abuse on children: A review and synthesis of recent empirical studies. *Psychological Bulletin, 113*, 164–180.

Keyser, J. L., Seelaus, K., & Kahan, G. B. (2000). Children's trauma and loss: Their treatment in group psychotherapy. In R. H. Klein & V. L. Schermer (Eds.), *Group therapy for psychological trauma* (pp. 209–238). New York: Guilford Press.

King, N., Hamilton, D., & Ollendick, T. (1988). *Children's phobias: A behavioural perspective.* New York: Wiley.

Knell, S. M. (1993). *Cognitive behavioral play therapy.* Northvale, NJ: Jason Aronson.

Kohlberg, L. & Ullian, D. Z. (1974). Stages in development of psychosexual concepts and attitudes. In R. C. Friedman, R. M. Richart, & R. L. VandlWiele (Eds.), *Sex differences in behavior.* New York: Wiley.

Kopp, R. R. (1995). *Metaphor therapy: Using client-generated metaphors in psychotherapy*. New York: Brunner/Mazel.

Kovacs, M. (1989). Affective disorders in children and adolescents. *American Psychologist, 44*, 209–215.

Kratochwill, T. R. & Morris, R. J. (1993). *Handbook of psychotherapy with children and adolescents*. Boston: Allyn & Bacon.

Kristensen, H. (2000). Selective mutism and comorbidity with developmental disorder/delay, anxiety disorder, and elimination disorder. *Journal of the American Academy of Child and Adolescent Psychiatry, 39*, 249–256.

Kussmaul, A. (1877). *Die stbrugen der sprach*. Leipzig: PCW.

Lakoff, G. & Johnson, M. (1980). *Metaphors we live by*. Chicago: University of Chicago Press.

Langer, E. J. (1983). *The psychology of control*. Beverly Hills: Sage.

Lapouse, R. & Monk, M. A. (1958). An epidemiologic study of behavior characteristics in children. *American Journal of Public Health, 48*, 1134–1144.

Lazarus, A. (1984). *In the mind's eye: The power of imagery for personal enrichment*. New York: Guilford Press.

Lazarus, R. S. (1966). *Psychological stress and the coping process*. New York: McGraw Hill.

LeClerc, G. (1992). *Late-life potential*. Panel discussion presented at the annual meeting of the American Society on Aging, San Diego, CA.

Lefkowitz, M. M. & Burton, N. (1978). Childhood depression: A critique of the concept. *Psychological Bulletin, 85*, 716–726.

Leitenberg, H. & Callahan, E. J. (1973). Reinforced practice and reductions of different kinds of fears in adults and in children. *Behavior Research and Therapy, 11*, 19–30.

Lieb, R., Mastaler, M., & Wittchen, H. (1998). Gibt es somatoforme Stoerungen bei Jugendlichen und jungen Erwachsenen? (Somatoform disorders affect adolescents and young adults? First epidemiological findings based on a representative population sample). *Verhaltenstherapie, 8*, 81–93.

MacGregor, R., Pullar, A., & Cundall, D. (1994). Silent at school: Elective mutism and abuse. *Archives of the Disabled Child, 70*, 540–541.

Mahoney, M. J. (1983). Knowledge and power, privilege and privacy: Reflections on the boundaries of studying powerful persons and institutions. *Newsletter of the Society for the Advancement of Social Psychology, 9*, 16–22.

Mahoney, M. J. (1991). *Human change processes*. New York: Basic Books.

Mahoney, M. J. (1995). Continuing evolution of the cognitive sciences and psychotherapies. In R. A. Neimeyer & M. J. Mahoney (Eds.), *Constructivism in psychotherapy* (pp. 39–67). Washington, DC: American Psychological Association.

Manassis, K. (2000). Childhood anxiety disorders: Lessons from the literature. *Canadian Journal of Psychiatry, 45*, 724–730.

Mann, J. & Rosental, T. L. (1969). Vicarious and direct counterconditioning of test anxiety through individual and group desensitization. *Behavior Research and Therapy, 7*, 359–367.

Mark, R. S. & Douglas, U. (1999). The successful treatment of long-term selective mutism: A case study. *Journal of Behavior Therapy and Experimental Psychiatry, 30*, 313–323.

Marks, I. (1969). *Fears and phobias*. New York: Academic Press.

Marks, I. (1978). *Living with fear*. New York: McGraw-Hill.

Marks, I. (1987). *Fears, phobias and rituals*. New York: Oxford University Press.

Mash, E. J. & Barkley, R. A. (Eds.) (1996). *Child psychopathology*. New York: Guilford Press.

Mash, E. J. & Dozois, D. J. A. (1996). Child psychopathology: A developmental-systems perspective. In E. J. Mash & R. A. Barkley (Eds.), *Child psychopathology* (pp. 3–60). New York: Guilford Press.

Mash, E. J. & Terdal, L. G. (1988). Behavioral assessment of child and family disturbance. In E. J. Mash & L. G. Terdal (Eds.), *Behavioral assessment of childhood disorders* (2nd ed., pp. 3–65). New York: Guilford Press.

Maubach, D. M. (2000). The comorbid relationship of anxiety and depression in children and adolescents. *Dissertation Abstracts International [Section a: Humanities and Social Sciences], 60*, 3612.

May, R. (1975). *The courage to create.* New York: Norton.

McCloskey, L. A. & Walker, M. (2000). Posttraumatic stress in children exposed to family violence and single-event trauma. *Journal of the American Academy of Child and Adolescent Psychiatry, 39*, 108–115.

McNiff, S. (1992). *Art as medicine: Creating therapy of the imagination.* London: Butler & Tranner.

Meichenbaum, D. H. (1979). Teaching children self-control. In B. Lahey & A. Kazdin (Eds.), *Advances in clinical child psychology* (Vol. 2, pp. 1–30). New York: Plenum.

Meichenbaum, D. H. (1985). *Stress inoculation training.* New York: Pergamon.

Meichenbaum, D. H. & Goodman, J. (1971). Training impulsive children to talk to themselves: A means of developing self-control. *Journal of Abnormal Psychology, 77*, 115–126.

Meichenbaum, D. H. & Turk, D. C. (1987). *Facilitating treatment adherence: A practitioner's guidebook.* New York: Plenum.

Miller, S. H. (1979). Controllability and human stress: Method, evidence and theory. *Behaviour Research and Therapy, 12*, 287–304.

Minuchin, S., Baker, L., Liebman, R., Milman, L., & Todd, T. C. (1975). A conceptual model of psychosomatic illness in children. *Archives of General Psychiatry, 32*, 1031–1038.

Minuchin, S., Rossman, B. L., & Baker, L. (1978). *Psychosomatic families: Anorexia nervosa in context.* Cambridge, MA: Harvard University Press.

Moore, M. & Carr, A. (2000). Anxiety disorder. In A. Carr (Ed.), *What works with children and adolescents? A critical review of psychological interventions with children* (pp. 178–202). Florence, KY: Taylor & Francis/Routledge.

Morgan, R. T. T. & Young, G. C. (1975). Parental attitudes and the conditioning treatment of childhood enuresis. *Behavior Research and Therapy, 13*, 257–261.

Morris, R. J. & Kratochwill, T. R. (1983). *Treating children's fears and phobias: A behavioral approach.* New York: Pergamon Press.

Morris, R. J. & Kratochwill, T. R. (1991). Childhood fears and phobias. In T. R. Kratochwill & R. J. Morris (Eds.), *The practice of child therapy* (pp. 76–114). New York: Pergamon Press.

Mowrer, O. H. & Mowrer, W. M. (1938). Enuresis: A method for its study and treatment. *American Journal of Orthopsychiatry, 8*, 436–459.

Neimeyer, G. J. (1995). The challenge of change. In R. A. Neimeyer & M. J. Mahoney (Eds.), *Constructivism in psychotherapy* (pp. 111–126). Washington, DC: American Psychological Association.

Neimeyer, R. A. (1995a). An appraisal of constructivist psychotherapies: Contexts and challenges. In M. J. Mahoney (Ed.), *Cognitive and constructive psychotherapies: Theory, research and practice* (pp. 164–165). New York: Springer.

Neimeyer, R. A. (1995b). An invitation to constructivist psychotherapies. In R. A. Neimeyer & M. J. Mahoney (Eds.), *Constructivism in psychotherapy* (pp. 1–8). Washington, DC: American Psychological Association.

Neimeyer, R. A. (1995c). Constructivist psychotherapies: Features, foundations, and future directions. In R. A. Neimeyer & M. J. Mahoney, (Eds.), *Constructivism in psychotherapy* (pp. 11–38). Washington, DC: American Psychological Association.

Neimeyer, R. A. & Mahoney, M. J. (Eds.). (1995). *Constructivism in psychotherapy.* Washington, DC: American Psychological Association.

Olds, L. (1992). *Metaphors of interrelatedness: Toward a systems theory of psychology.* Albany: State University of New York Press.

Ollendick, T. H. (1983). Reliability and validity of the revised fear survey schedule for children (FSSCR-R). *Behaviour Research & Therapy, 21*, 685–692.

Ollendick, T. H., Matson, J. L., & Helsel, W. J. (1985). Fears in children and adolescents: Normative data. *Behaviour Research & Therapy, 23*, 465–467.

Patterson, G. R. (1976). *Living with children.* Champaign, IL: Research Press.

Patterson, G. R. (1982). *Coercive family process: A social learning approach.* Eugene, OR: Castalia.

Pennebaker, J. W. & Skelton, J. A. (1978). Psychological parameters of physical symptoms. *Personality and Social Psychology Bulletin, 4*, 524–530.

Peuler, J. N. (1988). Community outreach after emergencies. In M. Zealand (Ed.), *Mental health response to mass emergencies: Theory and practice.* New York: Brunner/Mazel.

Piaget, J. (1924). *The language and thought of the child.* London: Routledge & Kegan Paul.

Powell, M. B. & Oei, T. P. S. (1991). Cognitive processes underlying the behavior change in cognitive behavior therapy with childhood disorders: A review of experimental evidence. *Behavioural Psychotherapy, 19*, 247–265.

Powell, S. & Dalley, M. (1995). When to intervene in selective mutism: The multimodal treatment of a case of persistent selective mutism. *Psychology in the School, 32*, 114–123.

Prior, V., Lynch, M., & Glaser, D. (1999). Responding to child sexual abuse: An evaluation of social work by children and their caretakers. *Child and Family Social Work, 4*, 131–143.

Pynoos, R. & Nader, K. (1988). Psychological first aid and treatment approach to children exposed to community violence: Research implications. *Journal of Traumatic Stress, 1*, 445–473.

Rahav, G. & Ronen, T. (1994). Children's perceptions of their behavior problems during the Gulf War. *Anxiety, Stress and Coping, 7*, 241–252.

Rappaport, L. (1993). The treatment of nocturnal enuresis: Where are we now? *Pediatrics, 92*, 465–466.

Rasmussen, L. A. (1999). The trauma outcome process: An integrated model for guiding clinical practice with children with sexually abusive behavior problems. *Journal of Child Sexual Abuse, 8*, 3–33.

Raviv, A., Keinan, G., Abazon, Y., & Raviv, A. (1990). Moving as a stressful life event for adolescents. *Journal of Community Psychology, 18*, 130–140.

Redd, G. (1963). Elective mutism in children: A reappraisal. *Journal of Child Psychology and Psychiatry, 4*, 99–101.

Redd, W. H., Porterfield, A. L., & Andersen, B. L. (1979). *Behavior modification.* New York: Random House.

Reid, J. B., Kavanagh, K., & Baldwin, D. (1987). Abusive parents' perceptions of child problem behaviors: An example of parental bias. *Journal of Abnormal Child Psychiatry, 15*, 457–466.

Rey-Sanchez, D. F., Samino-Aguado, F. J., Lorenzo-Bragado, M. J., Pendas-Campos, A., & Gutierrez-Casares, J. R. (1995). Antecedents familiares de enuresis en ninos enureticos [Family history of enuresis in enuretic children]. *Revista-de-Psiquiatria-Infanto-Juvenil, 3*, 164–168.

Ritter, B. (1968). The group desensitization of children's snake phobias using vicarious and contact desensitization procedures. *Behaviour Research and Therapy, 6*, 1–6.

Roberts, M. C. (1986). *Pediatric psychology: Psychological interventions and strategies for pediatric problems.* New York: Pergamon Press.

Robin, S. J. (1999). An exploration of a multimodal approach for treating selective mutism. *Dissertation Abstracts International.*

Ronan, K. R. & Deane, F. (1998). Anxiety disorders. In P. Graham (Ed.), *Cognitive-behaviour therapy for children and families* (pp. 74–94). Cambridge, UK: Cambridge University Press.

Ronen, T. (1991). Intervention package for treating sleep disorders in a four-year-old girl. *Behavior Therapy and Experimental Psychiatry, 22*, 141–148.

Ronen, T. (1992). Cognitive therapy with young children. *Child Psychiatry and Human Development, 23*, 19–30.

Ronen, T. (1993a). Adapting treatment techniques to children's needs. *The British Journal of Social Work, 23*, 581–596.

Ronen, T. (1993b). Decision making about children's therapy. *Child Psychiatry and Human Development, 23*, 259–272.

Ronen, T. (1993c). Intervention package for treating encopresis in a six year old boy. *Behavioural Psychotherapy, 27*, 259–272.

Ronen, T. (1993d). Self-control training in the treatment of sleep terror disorder: A case study. *Child & Family Behavior Therapy, 15*, 53–63.
Ronen, T. (1994). Imparting self-control in the school setting. *Child and Family Behavior Therapy, 16*, 1–20.
Ronen, T. (1995). From what kind of self-control can children benefit? *The Journal of Cognitive Psychotherapy: An International Quarterly, 9*, 45–61.
Ronen, T. (1996a). Constructivist therapy with traumatized children. *Journal of Constructivist Psychology, 9*, 139–156.
Ronen, T. (1996b). Self-control exposure therapy for treating children's anxieties. *Child and Family Behavior Therapy, 18*, 1–17.
Ronen, T. (1997a). Cognitive–behavioural therapy. In M. Davies (Ed.), *The Blackwell companion to social work* (pp. 202–213). Oxford: Blackwell.
Ronen, T. (1997b). *Cognitive–developmental therapy with children.* Chichester, UK: Wiley.
Ronen, T. (1998a). Direct clinical work with children. In K. Cigno & D. Bourn (Eds.), *Cognitive–behavioural social work in practice* (pp. 61–80). Aldershot, UK: Ashgate/Arena.
Ronen, T. (1998b). Linking developmental and emotional elements into child and family cognitive behavioral therapy. In P. Graham (Ed.), *Cognitive behavior therapy for children and families* (pp. 1–17). Cambridge: Cambridge University Press.
Ronen, T. (2001). Collaboration on critical questions in child psychotherapy: A model linking referral, assessment, intervention, and evaluation. *Journal of Social Work Education, 1*, 1–20.
Ronen, T. & Abraham, Y. (1995). The relative efficacy of retention control training (RCT) for the treatment of younger versus older enuretic children. *Nursing Research, 45*, 78–82.
Ronen, T. & Ayelet. (2001). *In and out of anorexia: The story of the client, the therapist, and the process of recovery.* London: Jessica Kingsley.
Ronen, T. & Rosenbaum, M. (1998). Beyond verbal instruction in cognitive behavioral supervision. *Cognitive & Behavioral Practice, 5*, 3–19.
Ronen, T. & Rosenbaum, M. (2001). Helping children to help themselves: A case study of enuresis and nail biting. *Research in Social Work Practice*, 11, 338–356.
Ronen, T. & Wozner, Y. (1995). A self-control intervention package for elimination of enuresis. *Child and Family Behavior Therapy, 17*, 1–20.
Ronen, T., Wozner, Y., & Rahav, G. (1992). Cognitive intervention in enuresis. *Child and Family Behavior Therapy, 14*, 1–20.
Ronen, T., Rahav, G., & Wozner, Y. (1995). Self-control and enuresis. *Journal of Cognitive Psychotherapy: An International Quarterly, 9*, 249–258.
Rose, S. D. & Edelson, J. L. (1988). *Working with children and adolescents in groups.* San Francisco: Jossey-Bass.
Rosenbaum, M. (1990). The role of learned resourcefulness in self-control of health behavior. In M. Rosenbaum (Ed.), *Learned resourcefulness: On coping skills, self-control and adaptive behavior* (pp. 3–30). New York: Springer.
Rosenbaum, M. (1993). The three functions of self-control behavior: Redressive, reformative and experiential. *Journal of Work and Stress, 7*, 33–46.
Rosenbaum, M. & Ronen, T. (1997). Parents' and children's appraisals of each other's anxiety while facing a common threat. *Journal of Clinical Child Psychology, 26*, 43–52.
Rosenbaum, M. & Ronen, T. (1998). Clinical supervision from the standpoint of cognitive-behavioral therapy. *Psychotherapy, 35*, 220–229.
Rosie, S. (2000). Individual treatments for children and adolescents with post-traumatic stress disorder: Unlocking children's trauma. In D. K. Nath (Ed.), *Post traumatic stress disorder in children and adolescents* (pp. 131–146). London: Whurr.
Rupp, S. N. (1999). Haloperidol for Tourette's disorder plus selective mutism. *Journal of the American Academy of Child and Adolescent Psychiatry, 38*, 7–8.
Russell, A. B. & Trainor, C. M. (1984). *Trends in child abuse and neglect: A national perspective.* Denver: American Human Association.

Rutter, M., Yule, W., & Graham, P. (1973). Enuresis and behavioural deviance: Some epidemiological considerations. In I. Kolvin, R. C. MacKeith, & S. R. Meadows (Eds.), *Bladder control and enuresis* (pp. 137–150). London: Heinemann.

Rychlak, J. F. (1968). *A philosophy of science for personality theory*. Boston: Houghton Mifflin.

Sahler, O. J. Z & McAnarney, E. R. (1981). *The child from three to eighteen*. London: Mosby.

Safran, J. D. & Segal, Z. V. (1990). *Interpersonal process in cognitive therapy*. New York: Basic Books.

Salvatore, G., Maddalena, C., Lucia, P., Guido, M., & Paolo, B. (1999). Selective mutism, speech delay, dysmorphism and deletion of the short arm of chromosome 18: A distinct entity? *Journal of Neurology, Neurosurgery and Psychiatry, 67*, 830–831.

Schaffer, H. R. (1990). *Making decisions about children: Psychology questions and answers*. Oxford: Blackwell.

Schaffer, H. R. (1996). *Social development*. Oxford: Blackwell.

Schroeder, F. E. & Kendall, P. C. (2000). Group and individual cognitive-behavioral treatments for youth with anxiety disorders: A randomized clinical trial. *Cognitive Therapy and Research, 24*, 251–278.

Scotti, J. R., Mullen, K. B., & Hawkins, R. P. (1998). Child conduct and developmental disabilities: From theory to practice in the treatment of excess behaviors. In J. J. Plaud & G. H. Eifert (Eds.), *From behavior theory to behavior therapy* (pp. 172–201). Boston: Allyn & Bacon.

Shapiro, T. (1995). Developmental issues in psychotherapy research. *Journal of Abnormal Child Psychology, 23*, 31–44.

Shirk, S. R. & Russell, R. L. (1996). *Change process in child psychotherapy*. New York: Guilford Press.

Siegel, L. J. & Richards, C. S. (1978). Behavioral interventions with somatic disorders in children. In D. Marholin (Ed.), *Child behavior therapy* (pp. 339–394). New York: Gardner Press.

Siegel, L. J. & Smith, K. E. (1991) Somatic disorders. In T. R. Kratochwill & R. J. Morris (Eds.), *The practice of child therapy* (pp. 222–256). New York: Pergamon Press.

Silverman, W. K., Ginsburg, G. S., & Kurtines, W. M. (1995). Clinical issues in treating children with anxiety and phobic disorders. *Cognitive and Behavioral Practice, 2*, 93–117.

Strauss, C. C. (1988). Behavioral assessment and treatment of overanxious disorder in children and adolescents. *Behavior Modification, 12*, 234–251.

Swell, K. W. (1995). Personal and construct therapy and the relation between cognition and affect. In M. J. Mahoney (Ed.), *Cognitive and constructive psychotherapies: Theory, research, and practice* (pp. 121–138). New York: Springer.

Taylor, D. W. (1972). Treatment of excessive frequency of urination by desensitization. *Journal of Behavior Therapy and Experimental Psychiatry, 3*, 311–313.

Taylor, P. D. & Turner, R. K. (1975). A clinical trial of continuous intermittent and overlearning "bell and pad" treatment of nocturnal enuresis. *Behavior Research and Therapy, 13*, 281–293.

Terwogt, M. M. & Olthof, T. (1989). Awareness and self-regulation of emotion in young children. In C. Saarni & P. L. Harris (Eds.), *Children's understanding of emotion* (pp. 209–237). New York: Cambridge University Press.

Thompson, R. A. (1989). Causal attributions and children's emotional understanding. In C. Saarni & P. L. Harris (Eds.), *Children's understanding of emotion* (pp. 117–150). New York: Cambridge University Press.

Thomsen, P. H., Rasmussen, G., & Andersson, C. B. (1999). Elective mutism: A 17 year old girl treated successfully with citalopram. *Nordic Journal of Psychiatry, 53*, 427–429.

Thorsen, C. E. & Mahoney, M. J. (1974). *Behavioral self-control*. New York: Holt, Rinehart & Winston.

Thyer, B. A. & Sowers-Hoag, K. M. (1988). Behavior therapy for separation anxiety disorder of childhood. *Behavior Modification, 12*, 205–233.

Tramer, M. (1934). Elective mutism bei kinden. *Z Kinderpsychiatr, 1*, 30–35.

Ullmann, L. P. & Krasner, L. (1975). *A psychological approach to abnormal behavior* (2nd ed.). Englewood Cliffs, NJ: Prentice Hall.

Varni, J. W., Katz, E. R., & Dash, J. (1982). Behavioral and neurochemical aspects of pediatric pain. In T. J. Coates (Ed.), *Behavioral medicine: A practical handbook*. New York: Plenum.

Velosa, J. & Riddle, M. A. (2000). Pharmacologic treatment of anxiety disorders in children and adolescents. *Child and Adolescent Psychiatric Clinics of North America, 9*, 119–133.

Wadsworth, M. E., Hudziak, J., Heath, A. C., & Achenbach, T. M. (2001). Latent class analysis of child behavior checklist anxiety/depression in children and adolescents. *Journal of the American Academy of Child and Adolescent Psychiatry, 40*, 106–114.

Walsh, B. (Producer) & Stevenson, R. (Director). (1997). *Mary Poppins* [Video film] (Available from Walt Disney).

Waslick, B. D., Walsh, B. T., Greenhill, L., Eilenberg, M., Capasso, L., & Lieber, D. (1999). *Journal of Affective Disorders, 56*, 227–236.

Webster-Stratton, C. (1982). Teaching mothers through videotape modeling to change their children's behavior. *Journal of Pediatric Psychology, 7*, 279–294.

Webster-Stratton, C. (1993). Strategies for helping early school-aged children with oppositional defiant and conduct disorders: The importance of home–school partnerships. *School Psychology Review, 22*, 437–457.

Weisberg, R. W. (1993). *Creativity: Beyond the myth of genius*. New York: Freeman.

Wenar, C. (1982). Developmental psychopathology: Its nature and models. *Journal of Clinical Child Psychology, 11*, 192–201.

Werry, J. S. & Quay, H. C. (1971). The prevalence of behavior symptoms in younger elementary school children. *American Journal of Orthopsychiatry, 47*, 136–143.

White, W. C. & Davis, M. T. (1974). Vicarious extinction of phobic behavior in early childhood. *Journal of Abnormal Child Psychology, 2*, 25–37.

Wiszinckas, E. (1982). Preparing children for situational crises. *Journal of Children in Contemporary Society, 14*, 21–25.

Wolf, D. A. (1988). Child abuse and neglect. In E. J. Mash & L. G. Terdal (Eds.), *Behavioral assessment of childhood disorders* (2nd ed., pp. 627–669). New York: Guilford Press.

Wozner, Y. (1985). *Shinui behitnahagut* [Behavior change]. Tel Aviv: School of Social Work.

Wright, L. (1977). Conceptualizing and defining psychosomatic disorders. *American Psychologist, 32*, 453–456.

Youngerman, J. (1979). The syntax of silence: Elective mute therapy. *International Review Psychoanalysis, 6*, 283–295.

Zelenko, M. & Shaw, R. (2000). Case study: Selective mutism in an immigrant child. *Clinical Child Psychology and Psychiatry, 5*, 556–562.

Zikis, P. (1983). *In vivo* exposure and response prevention for rituals and tics in an 11-year old girl. *Behavioural Psychotherapy, 11*, 75–81.

About the Author

Tammie Ronen, Ph.D., is a professor at the Bob Shapell School of Social Work, Tel Aviv University. She is the president of the Israeli Association for Behavior and Cognitive Psychotherapy. For many years, she has been treating children and parents in her private practice, while studying and teaching in the field of child therapy in general and self-control therapy in particular.

Dr. Ronen has presented her research and clinical observations internationally. She has written many papers and books, most recently *Cognitive Developmental Therapy with Children* published in 1997 by John Wiley, which has been translated into four languages, and *In and Out of Anorexia: The Story of the Client, the Therapist, and Recovery* written with Ayelet and published by Jessica Kingsley in 2001.

Index